Color Atlas of
The Eye and Systemic Disease

© E E Kritzinger and B E Wright, 1984

This book is copyrighted in England and may not be
reproduced by any means in whole or part.
Distributed in North America and Canada by
Year Book Medical Publishers, Inc.
by arrangement with Wolfe Medical Publications Ltd.

Library of Congress Cataloging in Publication Data

Kritzinger, Erna E.
  A colour atlas of the eye and systemic disease.

    Bibliography: p.
    Includes index.
   1. Ocular manifestations of general diseases – Atlases.
I. Wright, Barry E. II. Title. III. Title: The eye and systemic
disease. [DNLM: 1. Eye manifestations – Atlases. WW 17 K92c]
RC73.5.K73   1984   616.07′5   83-26119
International Standard Book Number: ISBN 0-8151-5171-3

Printed by Royal Smeets Offset b.v., Weert, Netherlands

Color Atlas of

The Eye and Systemic Disease

Erna E Kritzinger   MSc, FRCS, MRCP

Consultant Ophthalmologist,
Birmingham and Midland Eye Hospital
and Selly Oak Hospital, Birmingham, England,
Senior Clinical Lecturer in Ophthalmology,
Medical School, University of Birmingham

Barry E Wright   MD, FACS

Associate Director, Retina Service,
Montefiore Hospital and Medical Center,
New York, USA,
Associate Professor in Ophthalmology,
Albert Einstein College of Medicine,
Yeshiva University, New York

Year Book Medical Publishers, Inc
35 East Wacker Drive, Chicago

We thank Heather M Beaumont, BSc, PhD, who compiled the index and assisted with the preparation of the manuscript.

Contents

	Page
Introduction	7
1 Inborn errors of metabolism	9
2 Inherited disorders involving the connective tissues	15
3 Acquired diseases of joints and connective tissues	19
4 Infections, infestations and granulomas	27
5 Dermatological disorders	37
6 Endocrine disorders	40
7 Cardiovascular and pulmonary disorders	48
8 Renal disorders	52
9 Haemopoetic and lymphoreticular disorders	53
10 Gastrointestinal and hepatobiliary disorders	57
11 Neurological and muscle disorders	58
Index	68

To our patients

Introduction

This Atlas aims to illustrate abnormalities of the eye associated with common systemic diseases. In addition it demonstrates some of the 'classic' eye signs of rarer disorders which all physicians are expected to recognise, but seldom have the opportunity to encounter.

Although designed primarily as an aid for those engaged in postgraduate studies in ophthalmology and internal medicine, it also provides a refresher course for clinicians already established in these specialities and in allied disciplines such as rheumatology, dermatology, endocrinology and neurology.

Erna E Kritzinger
Barry E Wright

1: Inborn errors of metabolism

Of the many inherited metabolic disorders with associated ocular signs, those occuring in Wilson's disease are among the few which provide the basis for a specific diagnosis. Abnormal amino acid metabolism is represented by homocystinuria and albinism and abnormal carbohydrate metabolism by galactosaemia.

Disorders of lipid and lipoprotein metabolism are among those most frequently presenting with ocular abnormalities and these are illustrated by hyperlipidaemia. The metabolic factors underlying retinitis pigmentosa remain to be elucidated although, in some instances, Vitamin A deficiency is implicated.

Wilson's disease (hepatolenticular degeneration)

In this metabolic disorder, transmitted as an autosomal recessive trait, there is a deficiency of the copper-binding plasma protein ceruloplasmin, resulting in deposition of copper in the brain, liver, kidneys and eyes.

The ocular abnormalities include a Kayser-Fleischer ring in the cornea and 'sunflower' cataract; both are pathognomic of Wilson's disease.

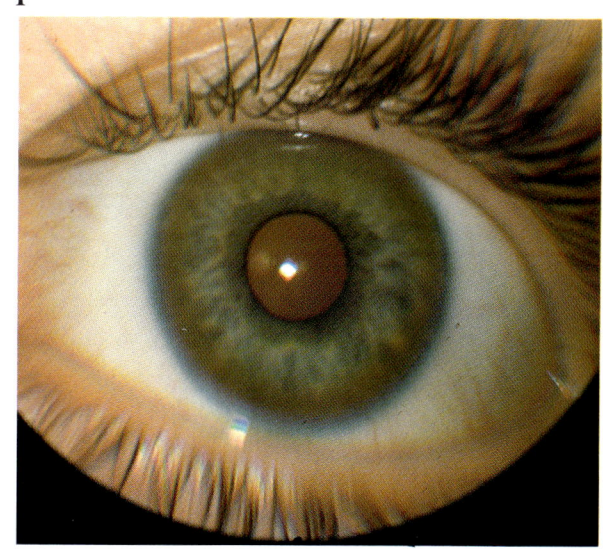

1 A Kayser-Fleischer ring. This is brought about by deposits of copper in Descemet's membrane, and is seen as a rusty brown ring at the corneal periphery.

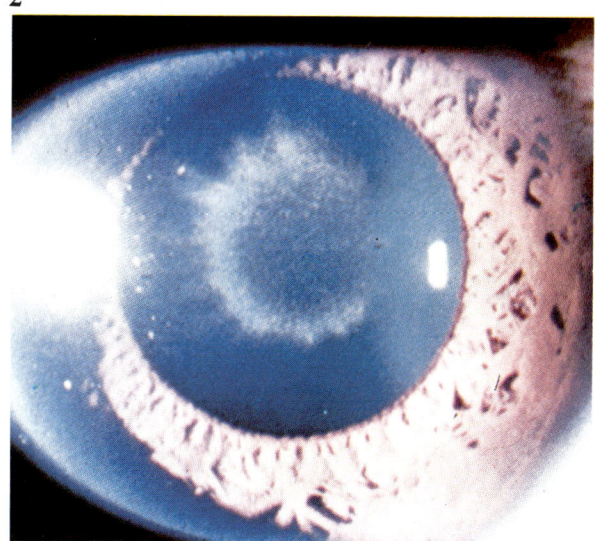

2 'Sunflower' cataract. Deposits of copper hydrate form a radiating pattern on the anterior capsule of the lens; normally vision is not seriously affected.

Homocystinuria

This is a metabolic disorder of amino acid metabolism in which deficiency of the enzyme cystathionine synthetase affects the normal formation of connective tissue and leads to an accumulation of homocystine in the blood and urine and methionine in the blood: it is transmitted as an autosomal recessive trait.

The patients, about 50 per cent of whom are mentally retarded, show skeletal and ocular changes similar to those occurring in Marfan's syndrome (page 15) from which homocystinuria has to be differentiated.

Dislocation of the lens (ectopia lentis) is a common presenting feature of both conditions. In homocystinuria the lens typically dislocates infero-nasally and may enter the anterior chamber of the eye. The dislocated lens predisposes to secondary glaucoma and retinal detachment and frequently becomes cataractous. Other ocular abnormalities include myopia, congenital glaucoma (buphthalmos), peripheral retinal degeneration and optic atrophy.

Thromboembolic disease is an additional factor associated with homocystinuria, and makes ophthalmic surgery hazardous.

3 Ectopia lentis in homocystinuria. The lens has dislocated into the anterior chamber of the eye and lies in front of the pupil. (Illustration by courtesy of Miss E M Eagling.)

Albinism

There are three types of albinism, all of them caused by abnormal melanin production.

Oculocutaneous (tyrosine negative) albinism is caused by absence of the enzyme tyrosinase, blocking the conversion of tyrosine to dopa in the biosynthesis of melanin. This is the most extreme form of albinism, individuals being characterised by white hair, pink skin and cutaneous photosensitivity. The irides are blue-grey and diaphanous, the retinal red reflex is prominent and the fundus lacks pigment. Visual acuity is reduced due to photophobia, hypermetropia and a high degree of astigmatism. Nystagmus is common.

Oculocutaneous (tyrosine positive) albinism resembles the tyrosine negative form of the disease in that it is carried as an autosomal recessive trait; individuals have normal levels of tyrosine, however, and are less affected. Skin, hair and ocular pigmentation increase with age. Visual acuity is moderately reduced because of photophobia and nystagmus but tends to improve throughout childhood.

Ocular albinism may be inherited either as an X-linked or autosomal recessive character and affects the eyes only. The clinical signs are similar to those described for tyrosine negative oculocutaneous albinism; although the irides may be pigmented, visual acuity is reduced. Visual acuity is normal in female carriers of the disease, but they have diaphanous irides and pigmentary abnormalities of the retina.

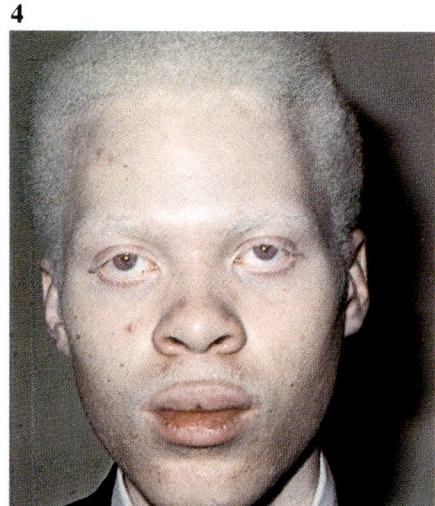

4 **Oculocutaneous (tyrosine negative) albinism in a negro.**

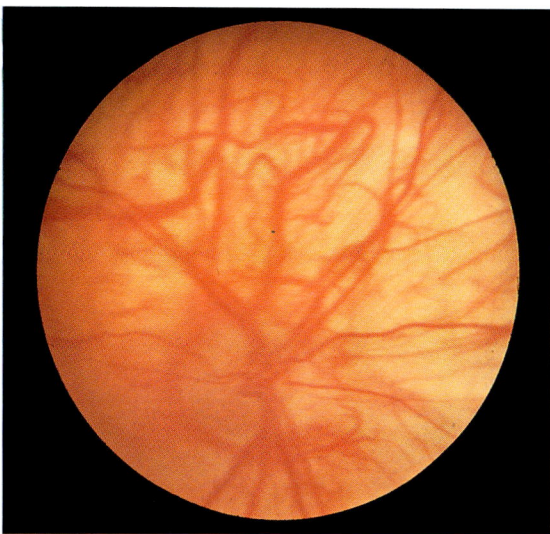

5 **The fundus in albinism** lacks pigment; retinal and choroidal vessels show up against the underlying white sclera.

Galactosaemia

There are two forms of galactosaemia, both of them autosomal recessive inherited abnormalities of carbohydrate metabolism.

In 'classic' galactosaemia, deficiency of the enzyme galactose-1-phosphate-uridyl-transferase leads to accumulation of galactose-1-phosphate and galactose in the blood and other tissues: cataract, mental retardation, hepatomegaly, jaundice and malnutrition result.

In the second, milder form of the disorder there is a deficiency of the enzyme galactose kinase which results in accumulation of galactose in the blood and other tissues. Cataract formation is the only clinical sign.

Individuals affected with either of these conditions may have cataracts at birth although, more frequently, they develop them within the first few weeks of life. Dietary elimination of galactose during early life may arrest cataractous changes or even bring about a regression.

6 **Cataract in galactosaemia.** The appearance is that of an 'oil drop' in the centre of the lens; zonular opacities may also occur. (Illustration by courtesy of Orthoptic Department, Children's Hospital, Birmingham.)

Hyperlipidaemia

In this disorder, abnormal plasma lipoprotein metabolism results in elevated plasma triglyceride and/or cholesterol levels. Friedrickson classified the condition into five types according to the levels of plasma lipoprotein: all of the types show ocular abnormalities (see Table).

In addition to the abnormalities tabulated, Type I shows xanthomata of the iris; Types III, IV and V show early atherosclerotic changes in the retinal vessels and also tend to develop diabetes mellitus with its associated ocular abnormalities (page 44).

Type	Eyelids	Cornea	Fundus
I	Eruptive xanthomata	Lipid keratopathy	Lipaemia retinalis; adult onset Coats' disease
II	Xanthelasmata	Corneal arcus	Lipaemia retinalis very rare
III	Eruptive xanthomata	Corneal arcus; crystalline corneal dystrophy	Lipaemia retinalis
IV	Eruptive xanthomata		Lipaemia retinalis
V	Eruptive xanthomata		Lipaemia retinalis; retinal vascular occlusion

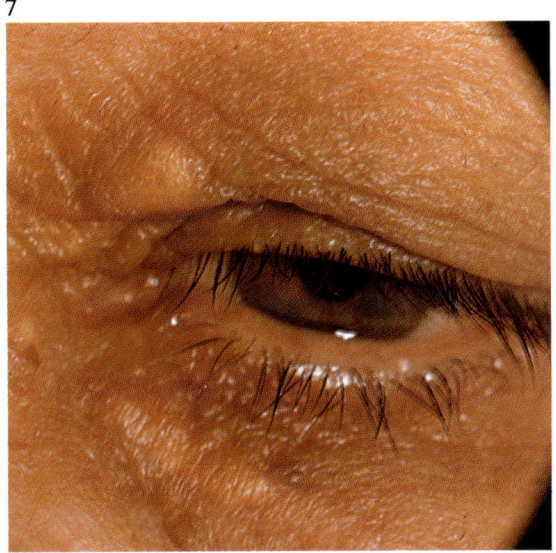

7 Xanthelasmata. Deposits of lipid material appear as yellow plaques on the skin of the eyelids, particularly towards the medial angle of the eye.

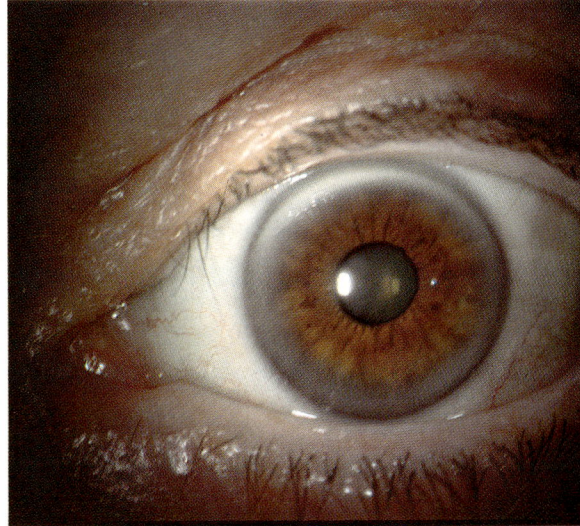

8 Corneal arcus. Deposits of phospholipid and cholesterol in the corneal stroma form a white ring at the corneal periphery with, typically, a concentric clear zone at its margin. This condition is a normal phenomenon associated with ageing (arcus senilis) but in patients under 50 years of age should alert to the possibility of hyperlipidaemia.

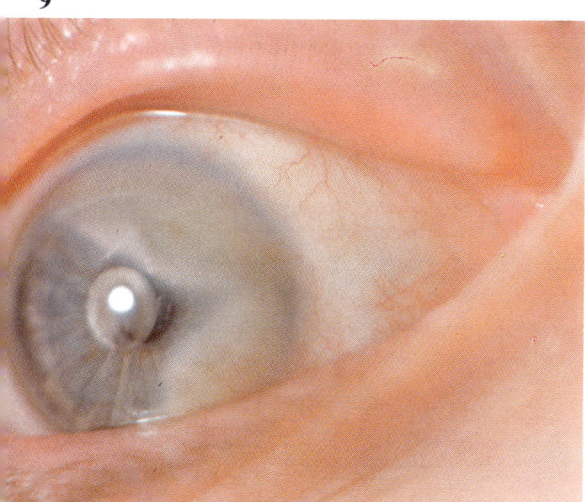

9 Lipid keratopathy. The corneal stroma is infiltrated by a lipid deposit which markedly affects vision.

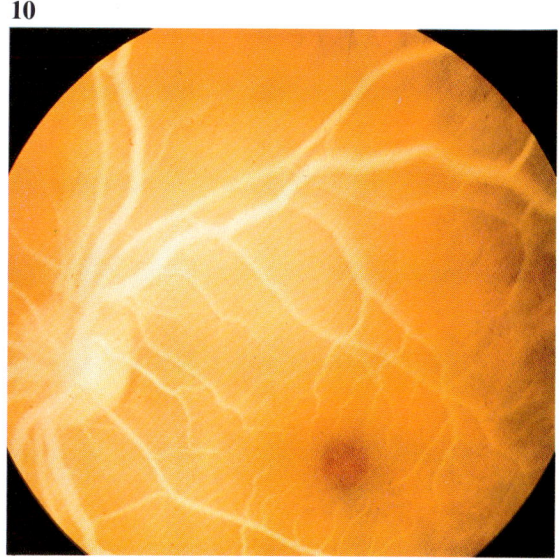

10 Lipaemia retinalis. This occurs when plasma triglyceride levels exceed 2,000 mg/ml. Vision is unaffected. Retinal vessels appear milky and engorged and stand out against the choroid. It also occurs, rarely, in patients with uncontrolled diabetes mellitus; it disappears with stabilisation of the diabetes.

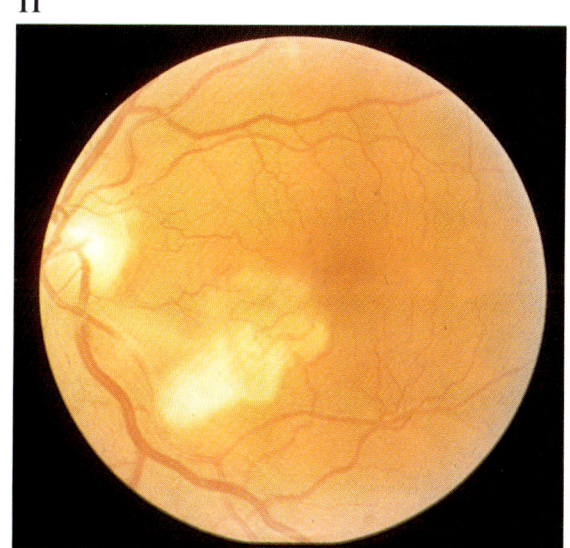

11 Retinal vascular occlusion. The inferior retinal branch arteriole is occluded and the infarcted retina is pale.

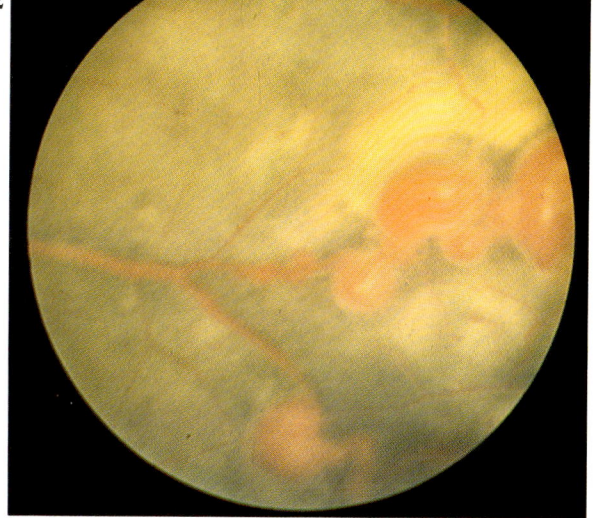

12 Coats' disease. Retinal telangiectasia occurs in the peripheral fundus with deposition of exudates in the surrounding retina. Exudative retinal detachment and thrombotic (neovascular) glaucoma are known complications. This condition usually occurs only in young children; it has been reported in association with hypercholesterolaemia in adults.

Retinitis pigmentosa

This term represents a primary degeneration of the retina, especially the photoreceptors, which may be inherited in any pattern.

Retinitis pigmentosa may present as an independent ophthalmological disorder leading to progressive loss of peripheral vision and night blindness. It may be accompanied by other ocular features including cataract, myopia, optic atrophy and attenuation of retinal vessels. Alternatively it may be part of a systemic disorder. Numerous syndromes have been described, in many of which the underlying metabolic disturbance still has to be elucidated. Examples include:

—retinitis pigmentosa with obesity, mental retardation, polydactyli, hypogonadism – Laurence-Moon-Biedl syndrome;

—retinitis pigmentosa with acanthosis of red blood cells, malabsorption of fats, spinocerebellar ataxia – Bassen-Kornzweig syndrome (abetalipoproteinaemia);

—retinitis pigmentosa with cerebellar ataxia, progressive peripheral polyneuritis – Refsum's disease (phytanic acid storage disease);

—retinitis pigmentosa and deafness – Usher's syndrome.

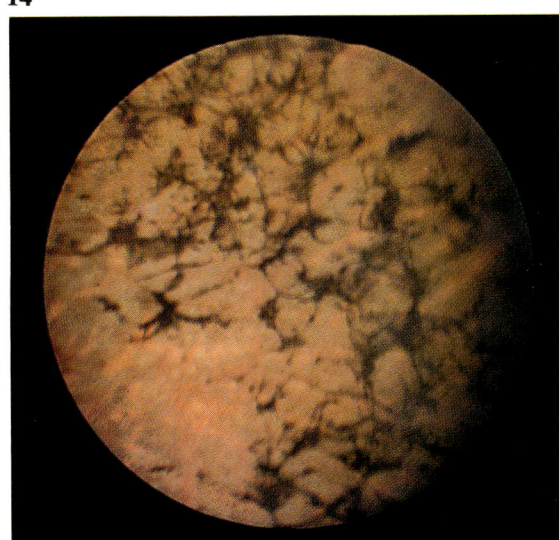

13 Retinitis pigmentosa. There are scattered areas of pigmentary degeneration in the fundus. The optic disc is pale and the retinal vessels attenuated.

14 'Bone corpuscle' configuration. This is characteristic of the retinal pigmentary degeneration in retinitis pigmentosa; the abnormal pigment overlies the retinal vessels.

2: Inherited disorders involving the connective tissues

In this group of disorders genetic defects in connective tissues involve multiple organ systems, including the eyes. Ocular abnormalities are associated with abnormal elastic tissue in Marfan's syndrome and Grönblad-Strandberg syndrome, with defective collagen in Ehlers-Danlos syndrome and with anomalies in the vascular supply to skin and mucous membranes in Rendu-Osler-Weber syndrome.

Marfan's syndrome

This autosomal dominant disorder of mesenchyme is expressed as defects in elastic tissue in the skeletal and cardiovascular systems as well as in the eye.

Patients have abnormal body proportions because of elongation of the long bones and laxity of the joints. Cardiovascular abnormalities include dissecting aortic aneurysm and mitral valve disease.

Ectopia lentis is the most common ocular abnormality and occurs in about 50 per cent of patients. The lens usually dislocates supero-nasally (cf homocystinuria, page 10) and frequently becomes cataractous; secondary glaucoma and retinal detachment may follow. Other ocular manifestations include blue sclerae, heterochromia of the iris, squint and myopia; colobomas of the lens, uvea and optic disc may also occur.

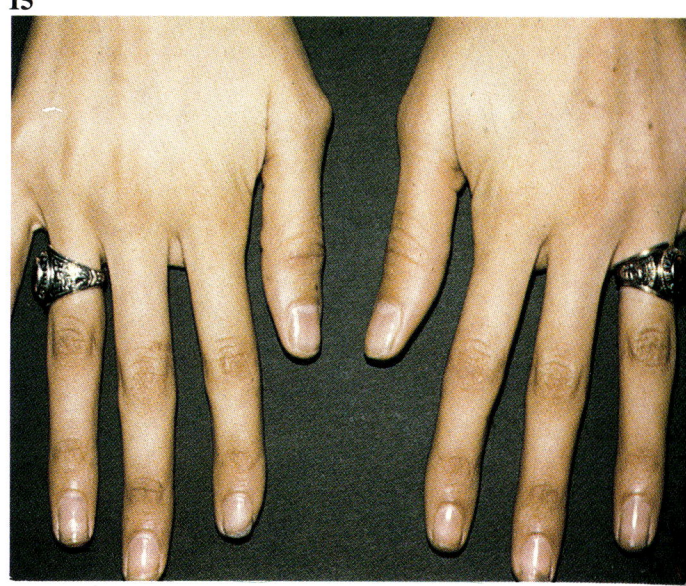

15 Arachnodactyli or 'spider fingers', caused by lengthening of the phalanges, are characteristic of Marfan's syndrome.

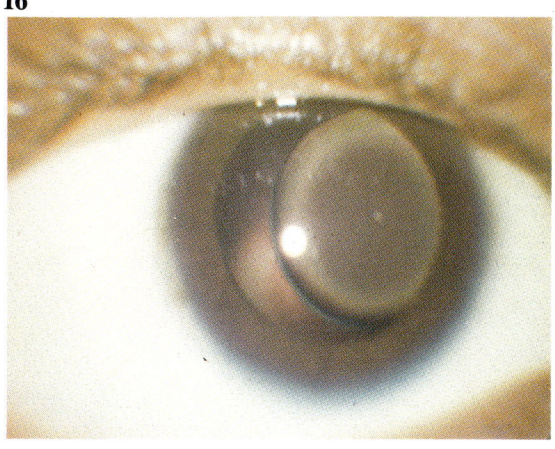

16 Ectopia lentis. The lateral border of the dislocated lens, displaced supero-nasally, is visible behind the pupil and a central lens opacity (cataract) is present. Dislocation of the lens may be demonstrated by tremor of the iris (iridodinesis) during movement of the eye.

Grönblad – Strandberg syndrome

The characteristic features of this syndrome involve the elastic tissues of the skin, eye and arteries: they include pseudoxanthoma elasticum of the skin, angioid streaks of the retina and systemic arterial abnormalities (occlusion, dilatation and haemorrhage).

Angioid streaks of the retina often present in the second or third decades by causing macular haemorrhages with scar formation. The retinal changes occur bilaterally and are slowly progressive, eventually causing central visual defects in 70 per cent of patients with Grönblad-Strandberg syndrome.

The syndrome may be inherited as an autosomal dominant or recessive trait.

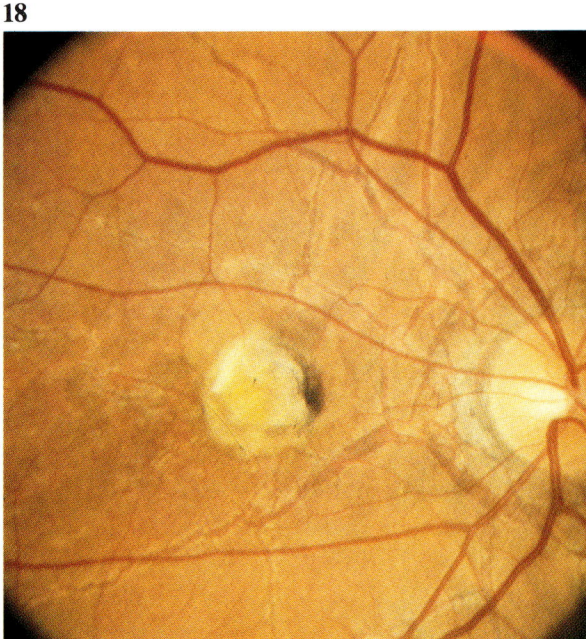

17 Pseudoxanthoma elasticum. There are yellow xanthoma-like papular skin lesions on the neck, where they are most commonly found. Other skin areas frequently involved include the skin creases of limbs, axillae and groin, and the peri-umbilical region.

18 Angioid streaks in the retina. These arise as a result of breaks in Bruch's membrane. They take the form of grey-brown branching streaks which seem to emanate from the optic disc, are irregular in outline and lie beneath the retinal vessels. A scar in the macula from previous subretinal neovascularisation is also apparent.

Angioid streaks in the retina are also found in cases of Ehlers-Danlos syndrome (page 17), acromegaly (page 41), Paget's disease, sickle cell anaemia (page 54), hypercalcaemia and lead poisoning.

Ehlers – Danlos syndrome

This generalised disorder of connective tissue may be inherited in one of several patterns; autosomal dominant, autosomal recessive or X-linked recessive. Hyperelasticity of the skin and hypermobility of the joints are characteristic features; recurrent dislocations of the joints are common.

Ocular manifestations include epicanthal folds, blue sclera, keratoconus, ectopia lentis, angioid streaks in the retina (page 16), and squint.

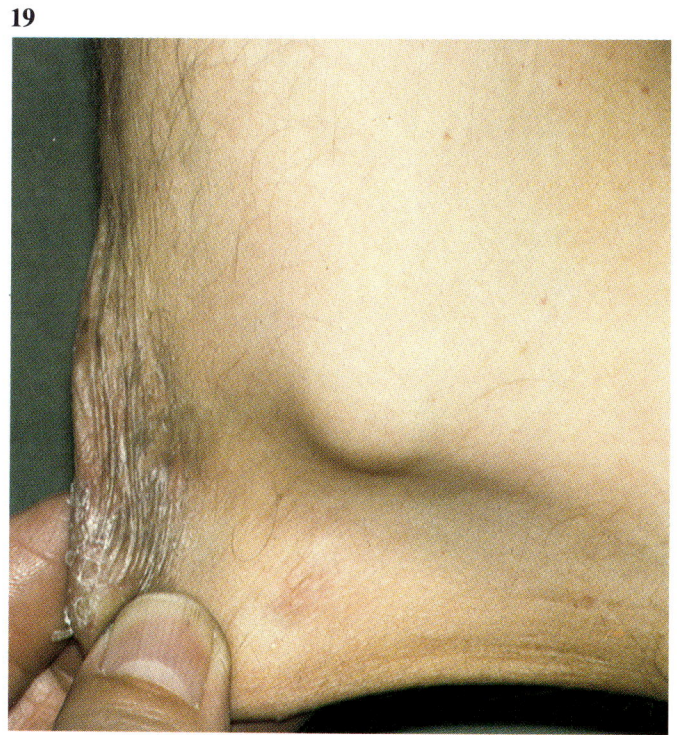

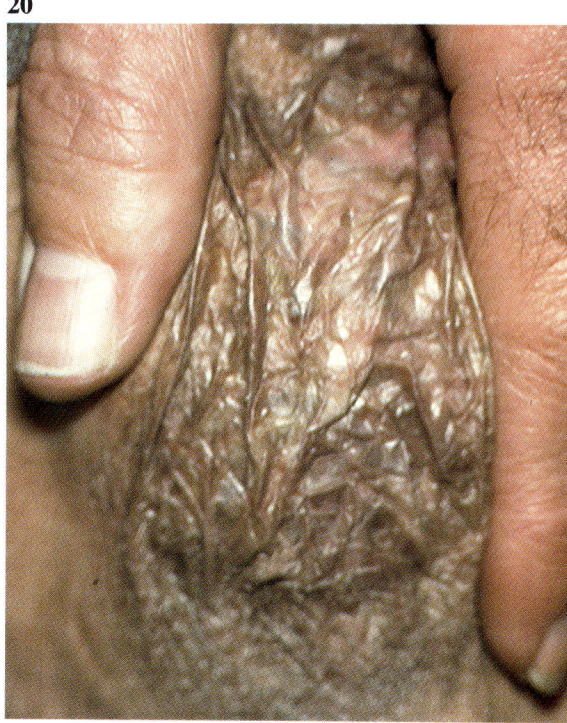

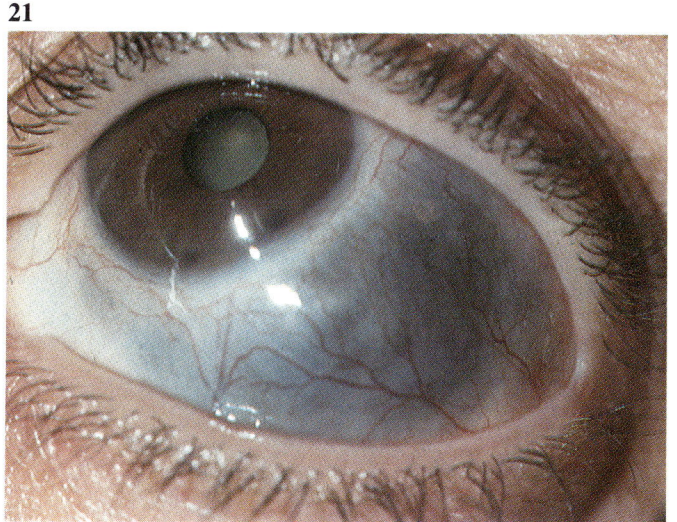

19 Hyperelasticity of the skin in Ehlers-Danlos syndrome.

20 The hyperelastic skin in Ehlers-Danlos syndrome is fragile and prone to bruising.

21 Blue sclera. The underlying dark choroid is visible through the thinned sclera; minor injury may rupture the eye.

Rendu – Osler – Weber syndrome (multiple hereditary haemorrhagic telangiectasia)

In this disorder, transmitted as an autosomal dominant character, multiple telangiectases in the skin and mucous membranes may result in recurrent haemorrhages so that individuals tend to develop iron deficiency anaemia.

Ocular abnormalities typically involve the conjunctiva. Intraocular lesions occur in less than 10 per cent of cases when retinal vessels are affected, appearing tortuous and dilated. Neovascularisation of the retina and optic disc may lead to retinal and vitreous haemorrhage.

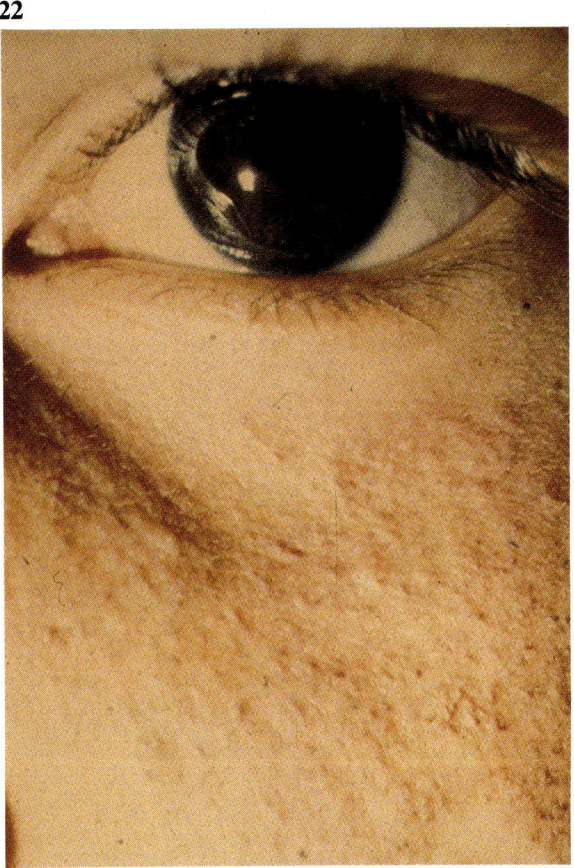

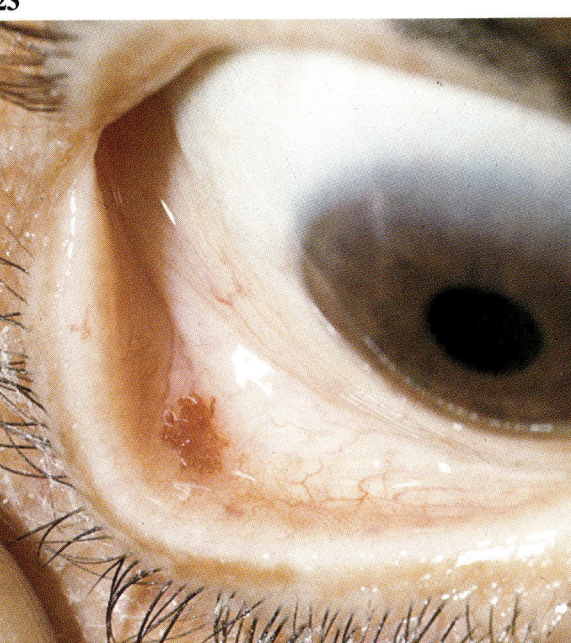

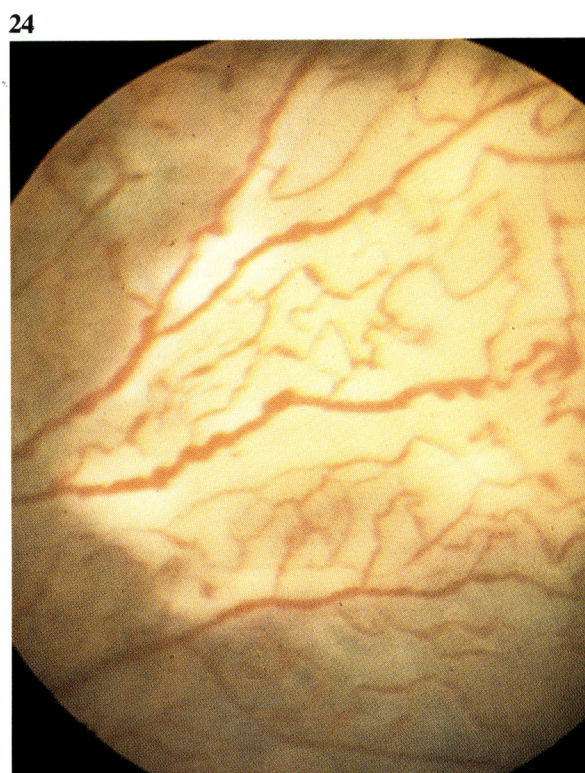

22 Multiple haemorrhagic telangiectases of the facial skin.

23 Conjunctival telangiectases. These are typically 'star-shaped'. The tarsal (eyelid) conjunctiva is more commonly involved than the bulbar (globe) conjunctiva.

24 Telangiectasia of retinal blood vessels.

3: Acquired diseases of joints and connective tissues

Many of the rheumatic disorders and other forms of polyarthritis have ophthalmic involvement. Similarly, the vasculitis underlying connective tissue diseases, such as systemic lupus erythematosus and giant cell arteritis, frequently causes ocular complications. The ocular abnormalities associated with these types of systemic disease are similar and are shared by other forms of vasculitis which, therefore, are included in this section. Commonly occurring ocular features are: conjunctivitis, episcleritis, scleritis, anterior uveitis (iritis), posterior uveitis (choroiditis), cataract, glaucoma, and various forms of retinopathy. In view of their common distribution, the ocular manifestations of each disease have been listed and representative illustrations selected.

Joint disorders

Rheumatoid arthritis: keratoconjunctivitis sicca, episcleritis, scleritis, iritis, cataract, glaucoma.

Still's disease: iridocyclitis, calcific band keratopathy, cataract, glaucoma.

Rheumatic fever: choroiditis.

Ankylosing spondylitis: iritis, cataract, glaucoma.

Psoriatic arthropathy: iritis.

Reiter's syndrome: conjunctivitis, iritis, episcleritis, retinopathy, optic neuritis.

Gout: iritis, glaucoma.

Connective tissue disease and vasculitis

Scleroderma (progressive systemic sclerosis): scleroderma of the eyelids with telangiectasia and lagophthalmos, keratoconjunctivitis sicca, atrophy of iris stroma and dilator pupillae, ischaemic and/or hypertensive retinopathy.

Systemic lupus erythematosus: unilateral proptosis, periorbital oedema, exopthalmoplegia, diplopia, keratoconjunctivitis sicca, episcleritis, scleritis, iritis, retinal vasculitis with ischaemic retinopathy, hypertensive retinopathy, chloroquine toxic retinopathy (iatrogenic).

Polymyositis and dermatomyositis: heliotrope skin rash on eyelids, periorbital oedema, ptosis, exophthalmoplegia, diplopia, conjuctitivitis, episcleritis, iritis, ischaemic retinopathy.

Wegener's granulomatosis: proptosis, ptosis, episcleritis, scleritis.

Giant cell arteritis: exophthalmoplegia, diplopia, iritis, scleritis, ischaemic optic neuritis and retinopathy.

Takayasu's (pulseless) disease: amaurosis fugax, retinal vascular occlusion.

Behçet's syndrome: exophthalmoplegia, diplopia, iritis with hypopyon, retinal vasculitis, retinal vein occlusion.

Rheumatoid arthritis

This form of inflammatory joint disorder is often associated with keratoconjunctivitis sicca, episcleritis, scleritis and cataract.

Keratoconjunctivitis sicca (dry eyes) and xerostomia (dry mouth) form part of Sjögren's syndrome; additional features of the syndrome include enlargement of the lacrimal and salivary glands, dryness of mucous membranes of the nasopharynx and tracheobronchial tree, as well as abnormalities of the pancreas, biliary system and thyroid. Over half of patients with Sjögren's syndrome have rheumatoid arthritis: other causes include sarcoidosis (page 35) and lymphomas (page 56).

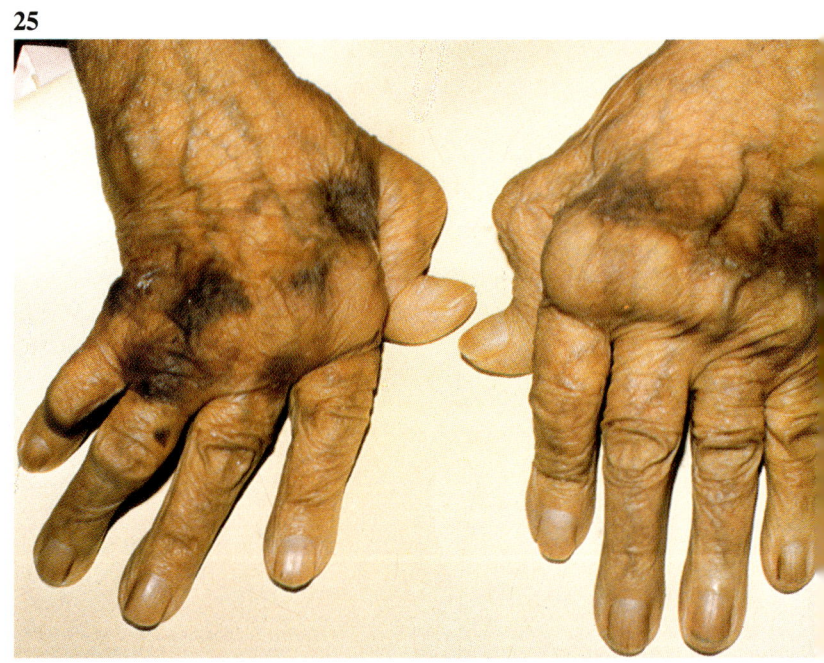

25 Rheumatoid arthritis of the hands.

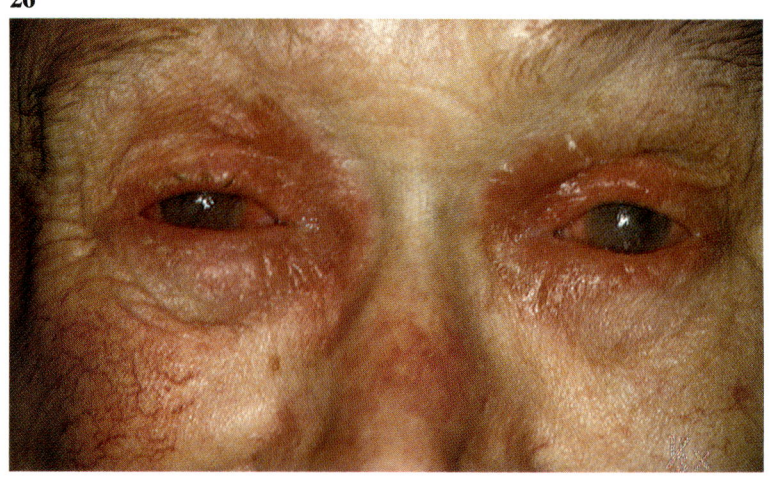

26 Keratoconjunctivitis sicca. The dry eyes are red and inflamed and both of the corneas show early scarring.

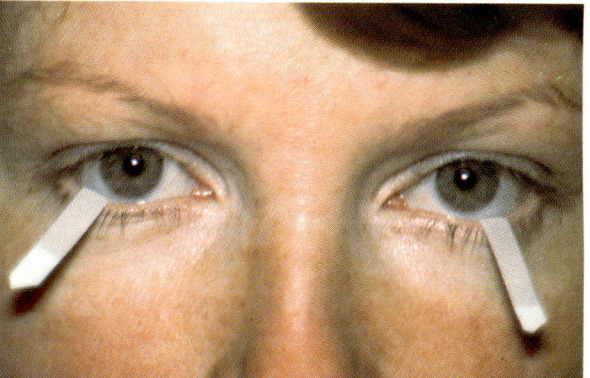

27 Schirmer's test for dry eyes. The volume of tear production is assessed by means of a strip of dry filter paper; wetting of less than 15 mm in 5 minutes is regarded as subnormal.

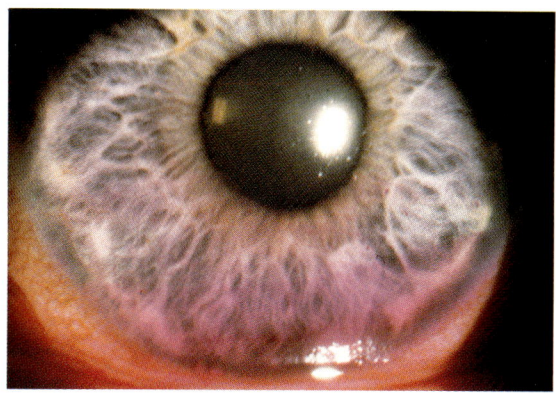

28 Bengal rose dye test for dry eyes. The red dye is taken up by desiccated epithelial cells in the cornea and conjunctiva.

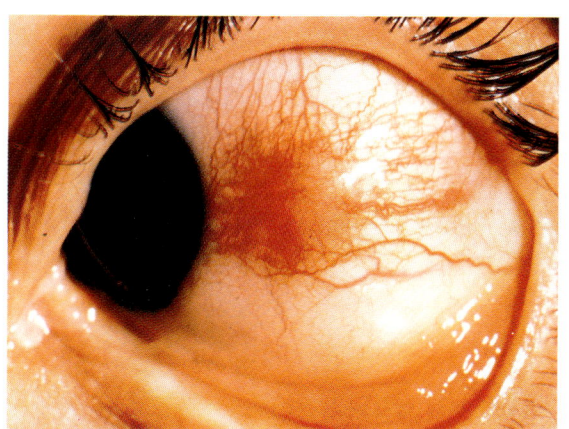

29 Episcleritis presenting as a localised and often painful area of inflammation lateral to the cornea. Inflammation of the episclera, the tissue which lies between the conjunctiva and the sclera, may also be a feature of infections and granulomatous disorders, eg tuberculosis, leprosy, syphilis, sarcoidosis (pages 28 and 35).

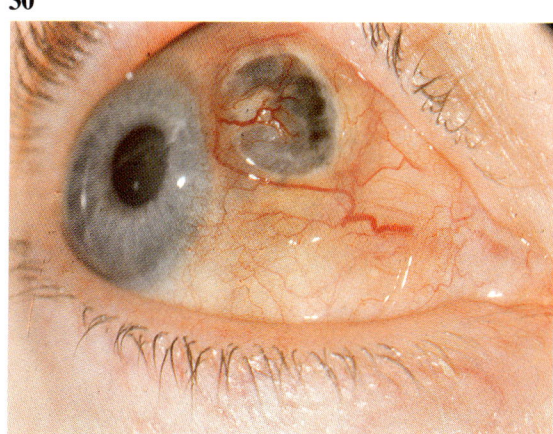

30 Scleromalacia perforans. Persistent scleritis with secondary thinning of the sclera have exposed the underlying choroid.

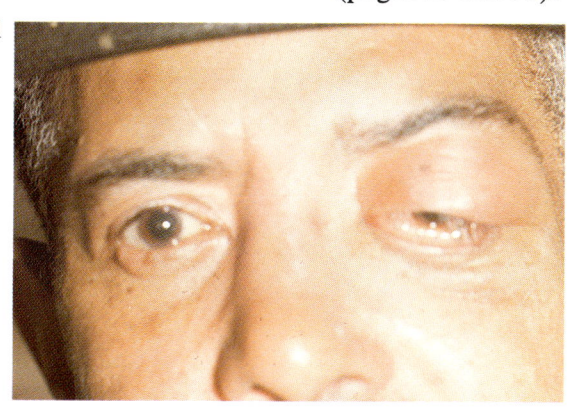

31 Proptosis. This may be a presenting feature of posterior scleritis. Related changes in the fundus include papillitis (page 58) and retinal oedema.

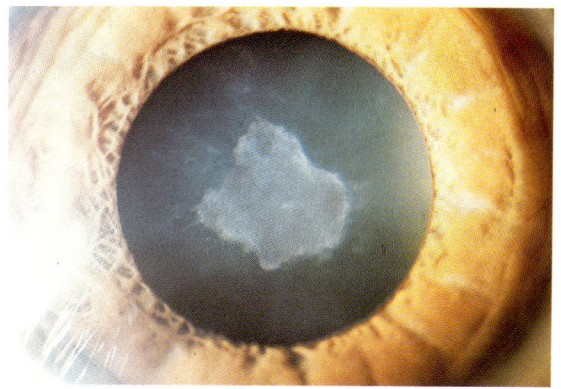

32 Cataract often occurs in patients with rheumatoid arthritis; it is usually caused by long-term treatment with systemic steroids.

Still's disease

Iridocyclitis (inflammation of the anterior uveal tract, involving the iris and ciliary body), which may be of insidious onset, is one of the most serious manifestations of this condition. When accompanied by calcific band keratopathy and cataract they form an ocular triad characteristic of Still's disease.

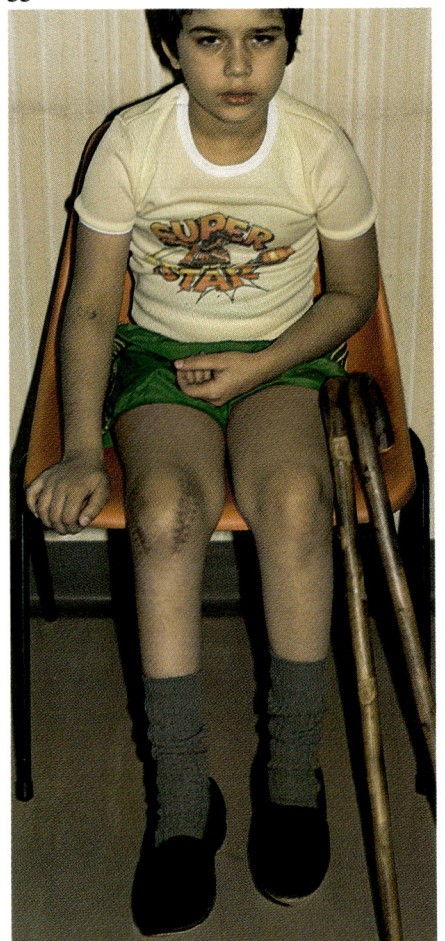

33 Still's disease. Both knee joints are affected.

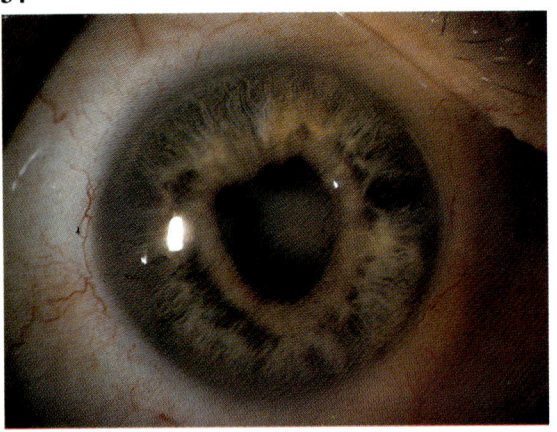

34 Iridocyclitis with a distorted pupil caused by adhesion of the iris to the lens (posterior synechiae).

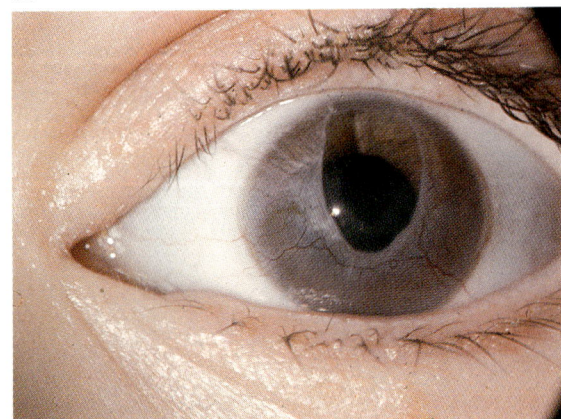

35 Calcific band keratopathy, secondary to iridocyclitis.

Reiter's syndrome

The three main features of this syndrome are non-bacterial urethritis, polyarthritis, and conjunctivitis or iridocyclitis.

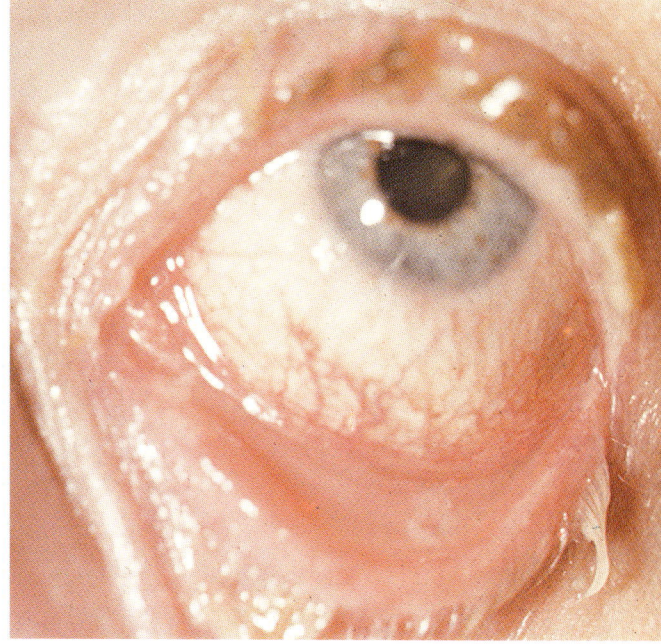

36 Conjunctivitis in Reiter's syndrome is mucopurulent in nature.

Gout

This is the term used to describe a heterogeneous group of disorders in which an increased serum urate concentration is associated with recurrent attacks of acute arthritis. A genetic predisposition is implicated in primary gout. In secondary gout, conditions leading to increased turnover of nucleic acids (e.g. myelo- and lympho-proliferative disorders, polycythaemia) or reduced renal excretion of urate (in renal disease) cause increased serum urate.

The ocular abnormalities include iritis and glaucoma.

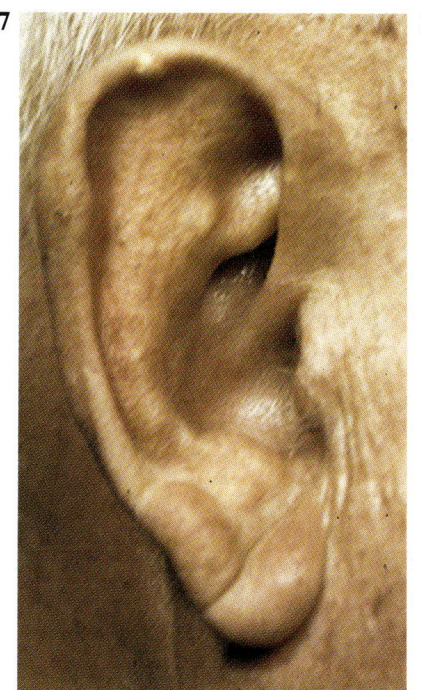

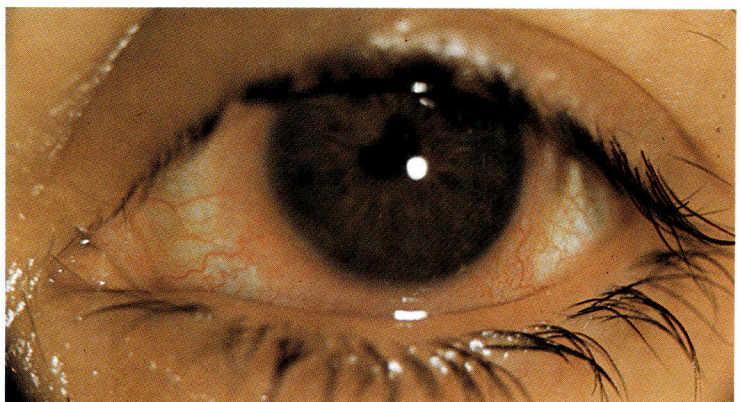

38 Gouty iritis. Onset is acute and painful. The pupil is small and irregular in outline because of the formation of posterior synechiae. Dilated blood vessels around the limbus of the cornea typically occur.

37 Gouty tophi on the helix of the ear. Crystals of monosodium urate are commonly deposited on cartilage.

Systemic lupus erythematosus (SLE)

This complex disorder is characterised by pronounced autoimmune phenomena and affects many tissues and organs in the body, including the eye.

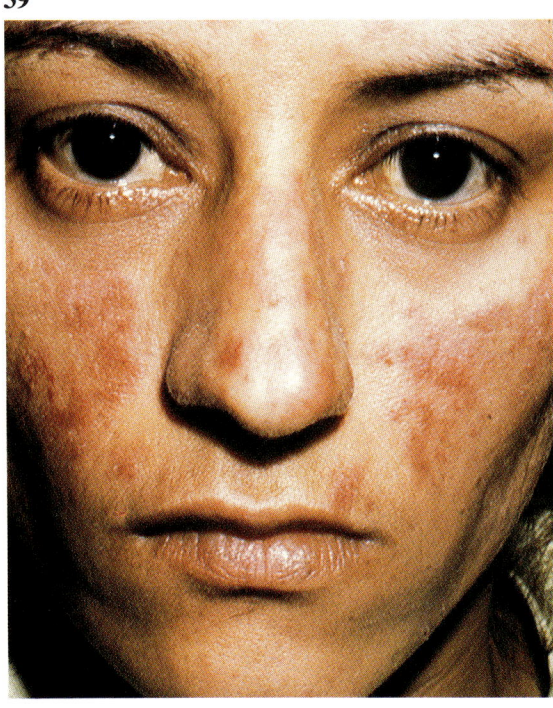

39 An erythematous 'butterfly' rash on the face is a classic sign in SLE.

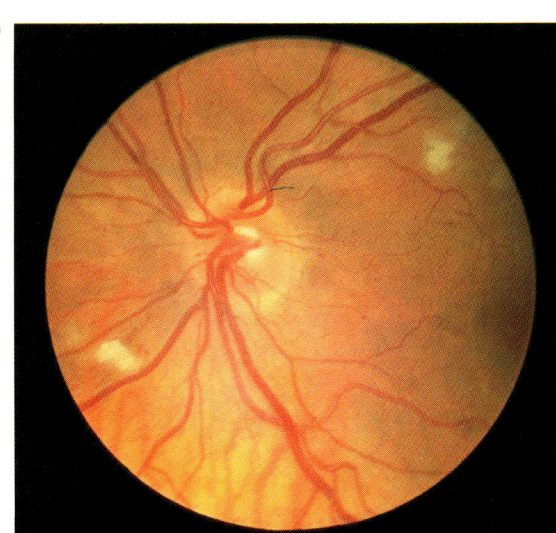

40 'Cotton-wool spots' in the fundus. These are caused by localised infarctions of the retinal nerve fibre layer and reflect severe retinal ischaemia. (See also pages 44, 48.)

41 Obliterative vasculitis. The retinal vessels are occluded and pale and there are retinal haemorrhages.

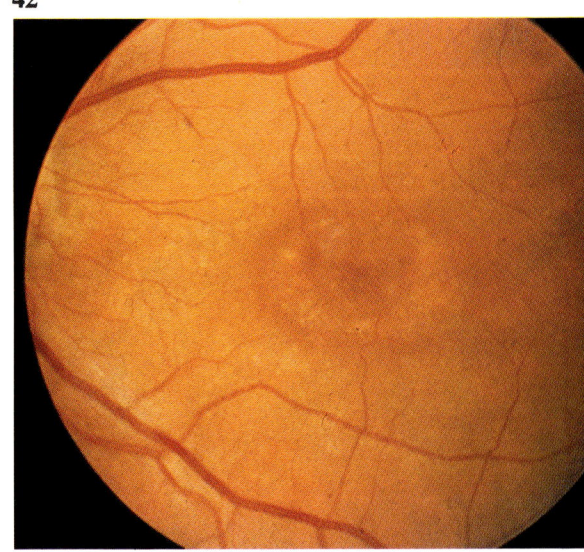

42 Chloroquine retinopathy. Chloroquine toxicity causes a typical 'bull's – eye macula' because of damage to the retinal pigment epithelium; central vision is severely affected. This is an iatrogenic hazard of chloroquine therapy for SLE.

Giant cell arteritis

A wide variety of systemic and ocular abnormalities occur in this inflammatory disorder of large and medium-sized arteries. A very high erythrocyte sedimentation rate is a characteristic finding.

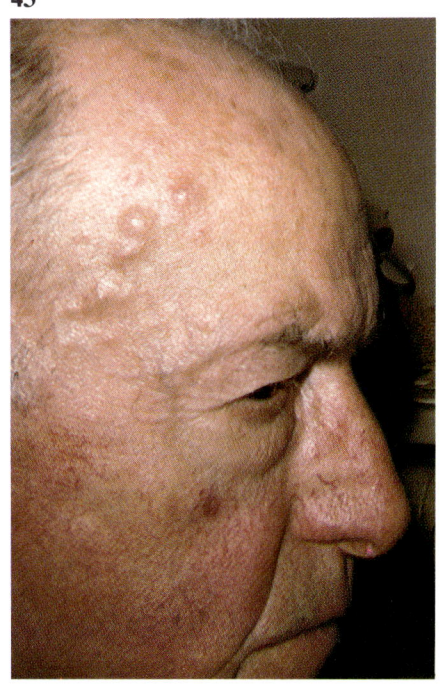

43 Giant cell arteritis involving the temporal artery. The nodular inflammation is painful and tender; biopsy of one of the nodules revealed multinucleate giant cells in the lamina elastica of the vessel wall.

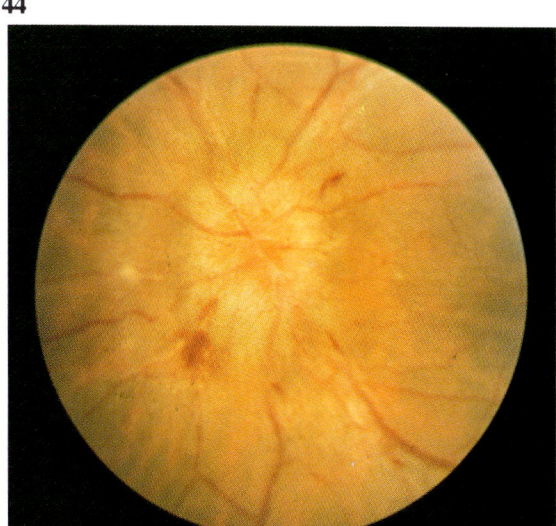

44 Ischaemic optic neuropathy caused by inflammation of the posterior ciliary arteries. The optic disc is pale and swollen and there is severe visual loss.

Takayasu's disease

This idiopathic inflammatory disease of large and medium-sized arteries causes progressive obliteration of the major branches of the aortic arch. Signs and symptoms of arterial insufficiency result, including a 'pulseless' state in the peripheral arteries. Amaurosis fugax may be a presenting symptom.

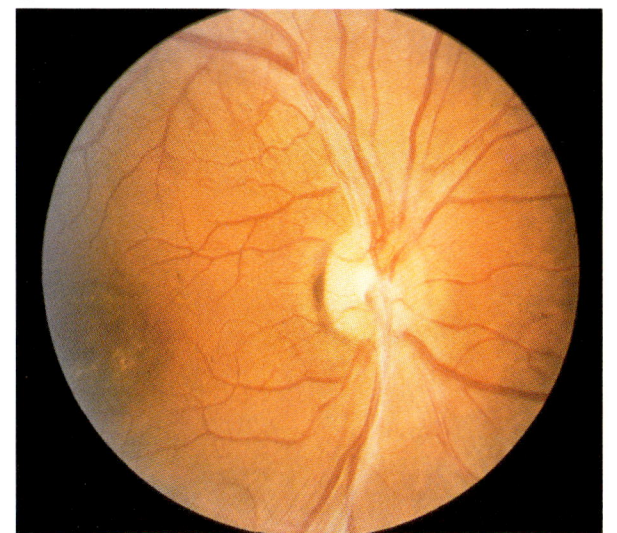

45 Takayasu's disease. There is occlusion of the central retinal artery.

Behçet's syndrome

The classic clinical triad associated with this chronic systemic inflammatory disorder includes ocular inflammation (anterior uveitis), recurrent aphthous-like stomatitis and genital ulceration. Other features include polyarthritis, thrombophlebitis, meningoencephalitis and skin lesions.

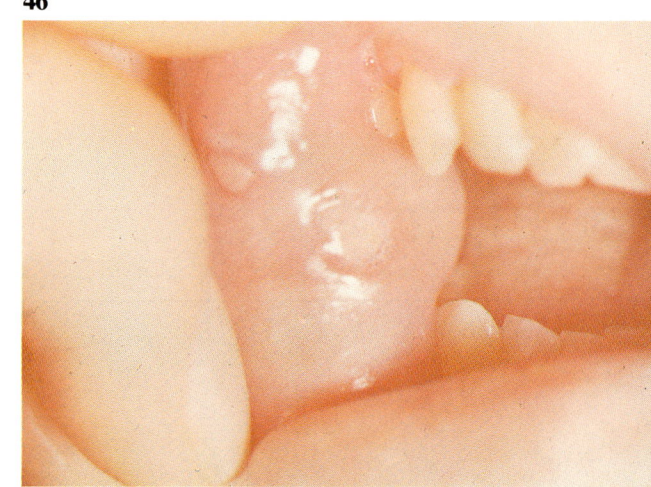

46 Ulceration of the buccal mucosa. This is a typical feature of Behçet's syndrome.

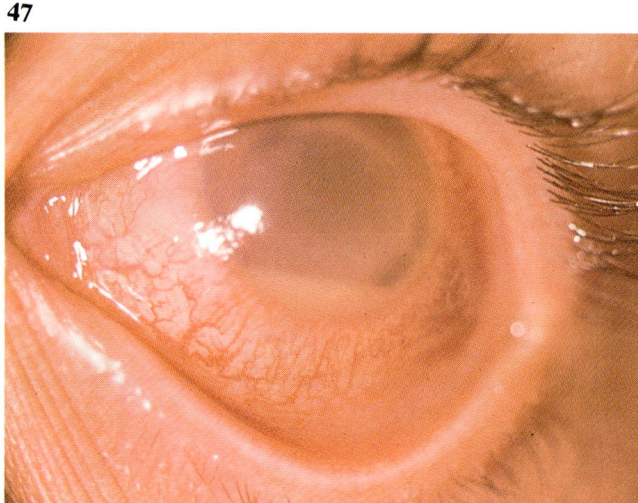

47 Hypopyon caused by severe recurring iritis.

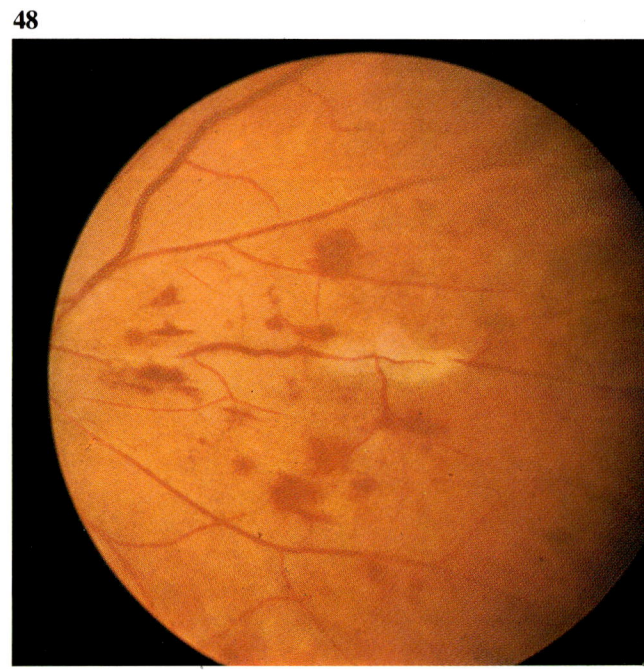

48 Retinal vein occlusion. This occurred secondary to periphlebitis.

4: Infections, infestations and granulomas

The eye may be involved in almost any type of systemic infection – bacterial, spirochaetal, viral, fungal or parasitic. Sarcoidosis, a granulomatous inflammation of unknown aetiology, is included in this section because of its similarities to tuberculosis.

BACTERIAL INFECTIONS
Bacterial septicaemia

Septic emboli from bacterial septicaemia may cause metastatic infections in the eye.

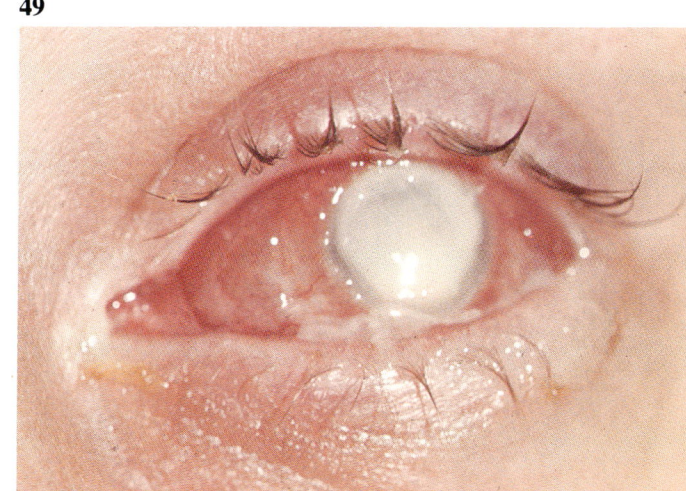

49 Septic endophthalmitis with necrosis of the cornea. The primary focus of infection was a staphylococcal furinculosis in a diabetic patient.

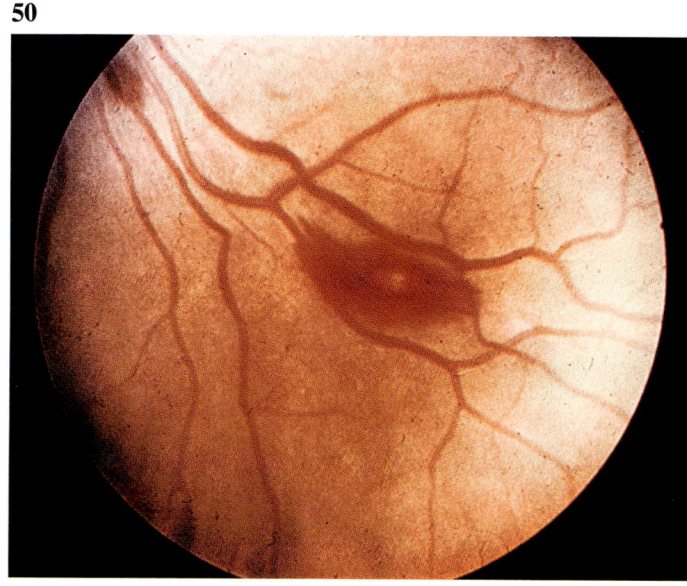

50 A septic embolus in a patient with subacute bacterial endocarditis has resulted in an oval haemorrhagic lesion with a white centre (Roth spot) in the retina. Roth spots are not pathognomic of bacterial endocarditis; they may also be found in anaemia and leukaemia (pages 53 and 56).

Tuberculosis

Ocular manifestations of tuberculosis include conjunctival ulceration, phlyctenular conjunctivitis, episcleritis, sclerosing keratitis, uveitis and choroidal deposits.

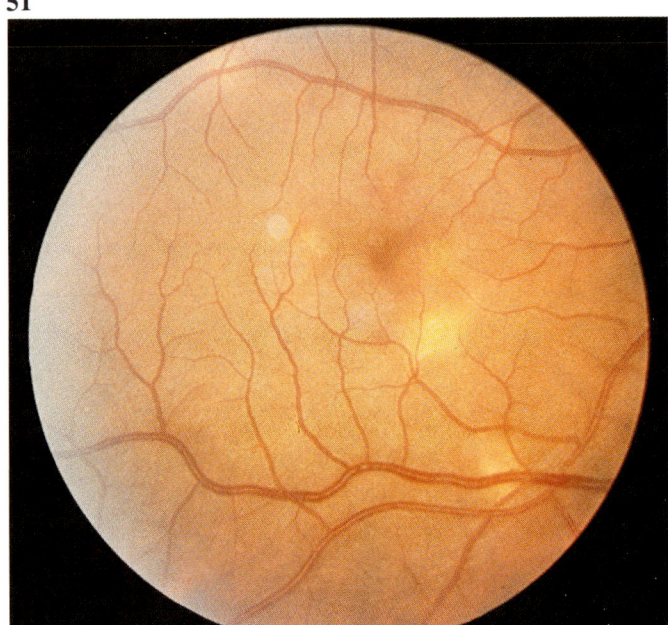

51 Miliary tuberculosis. Ill-defined pale tubercles are scattered in the fundus.

52 Choroidal tuberculoma. There is a pale cream tuberculous deposit temporal to the optic disc with a surrounding serous retinal detachment. Solitary choroidal tuberculomas are rare; when they occur they frequently show small, superficial haemorrhages. (The dark vertical line is a macular fixation target superimposed on the camera lens.)

SPIROCHAETAL INFECTION

Syphilis

Congenital syphilis may present with the following ocular features: interstitial keratitis, anterior uveitis (iridocyclitis), band keratopathy, secondary glaucoma, optic neuritis or atrophy, chorioretinitis ('salt and pepper' fundus), and chronic dacryocystitis.

Acquired syphilis may cause bilateral ptosis, Argyll-Robertson pupil, anterior uveitis, retinal vasculitis, chorioretinitis, optic neuritis and atrophy.

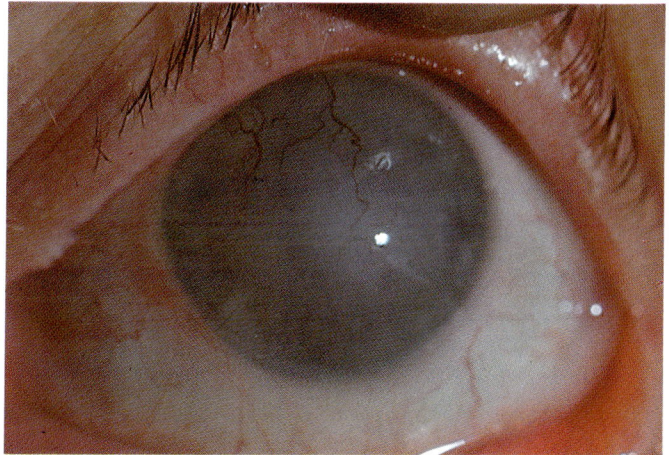

53 Interstitial keratitis. This has resulted in scarring of the cornea. Interstitial keratitis, eighth nerve deafness and deformity of the central incisor teeth are known as Hutchinson's triad in congenital syphilis.

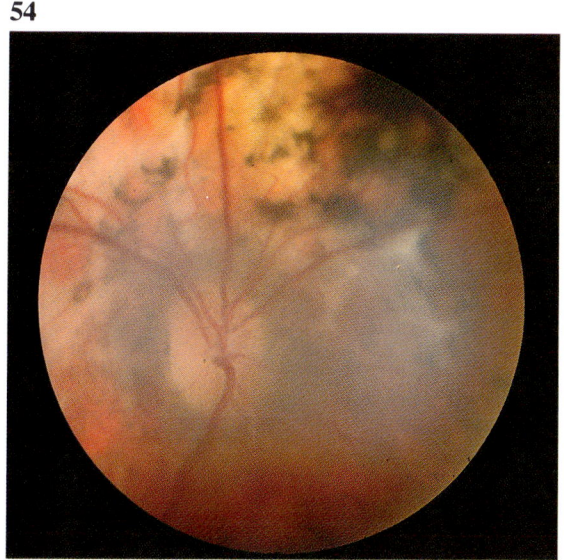

54 Chorioretinitis in acquired syphilis with diffusely scattered chorioretinal pigmentary scarring.

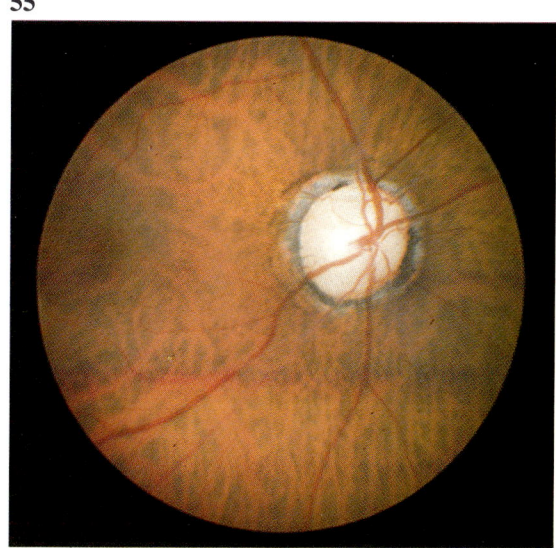

55 Optic atrophy in tertiary syphilis.

VIRAL INFECTIONS

Rubeola (measles)

In this infection, acute conjunctivitis and erosion of the corneal epithelium cause severe photophobia.

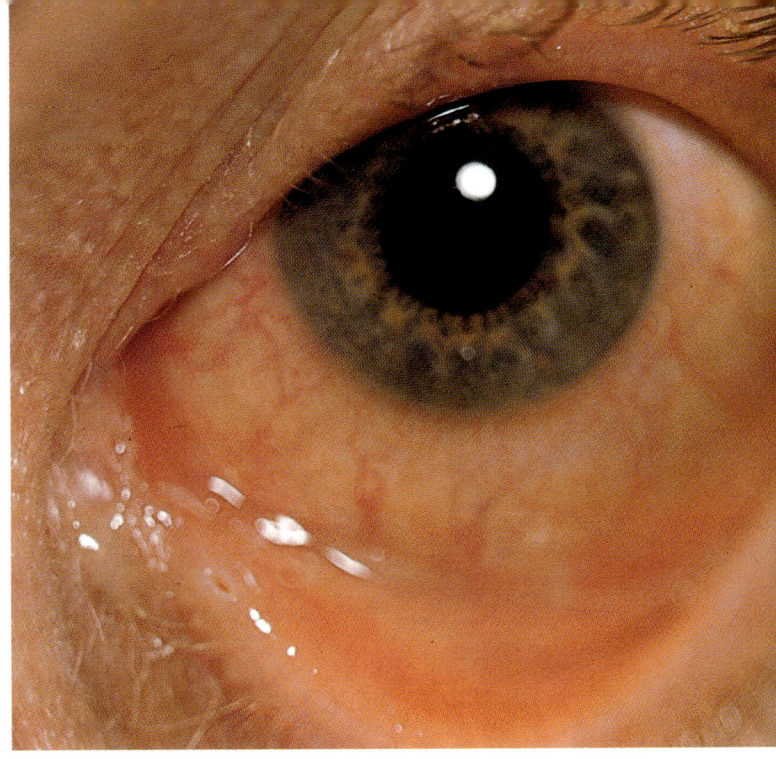

56 Conjunctivitis in measles. Both the bulbar (globe) and tarsal (eyelid) conjunctivae are involved.

Rubella (german measles)

Conjunctivitis is also commonly associated with rubella but, in contrast to that which occurs in measles, involves the bulbar conjunctiva only.

Maternal rubella during the first trimester of pregnancy results in a teratogenic intra-uterine infection and the congenital rubella syndrome. Ocular features of this syndrome include microphthalmia, cataract, glaucoma, uveitis, iris atrophy, and a 'salt and pepper' retinitis.

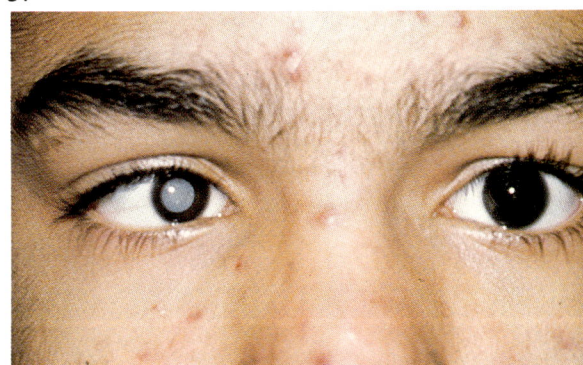

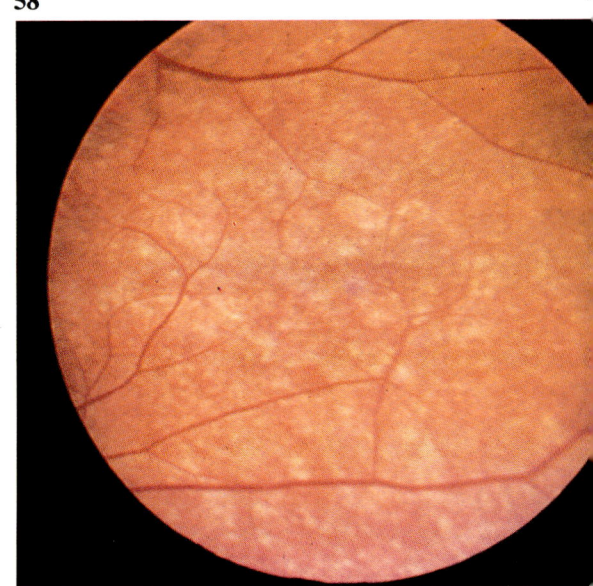

57 Congenital rubella with right microphthalmos, cataract and squint.

58 Rubella retinitis gives the fundus a 'salt and pepper' appearance.

Varicella – Zoster infections

The herpes virus, varicella-zoster, gives rise to two conditions:

Varicella (chickenpox) which may cause vesicular eruptions on the eyelids, conjunctiva and corneal limbus, occasionally associated with a mild keratitis and anterior uveitis (iritis).

Zoster (shingles) derives from a primary chickenpox infection involving the dorsal root or extramedullary sensory cranial nerve ganglia. Reactivation of the latent virus in the sensory ganglia gives rise to the clinical disease which may occur years after the primary infection. In the case of involvement of the trigeminal ganglion, vesicular skin eruptions appear in the dermatome supplied by the ophthalmic division of the fifth cranial nerve – hence the term 'herpes zoster ophthalmicus'. Ocular manifestations are common and may include:

Eyelids:	vesicular skin eruptions, blepharitis, cicatricial scarring with trichiasis
Extra-ocular muscles:	paresis, ophthalmoplegia
Cornea:	corneal opacities and infiltrates, corneal anaesthesia, ulceration and perforation (rare)
Conjunctiva:	conjunctivitis
Sclera:	scleritis
Lens:	cataract
Uvea:	uveitis with secondary glaucoma (20 per cent), iris atrophy with pupillary abnormalities, choroiditis
Retina:	necrotising vaso-occlusive retinitis
Optic nerve:	optic neuritis (rare)

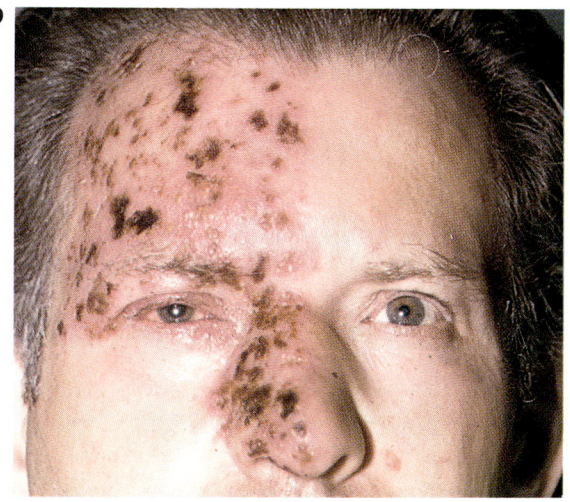

59 Herpes zoster ophthalmicus. The vesicular skin eruptions are in the distribution of the ophthalmic division of the fifth cranial nerve. Involvement of the tip of the nose which is supplied by the nasociliary nerve (Hutchinson's sign) indicates a high risk of ocular complications.

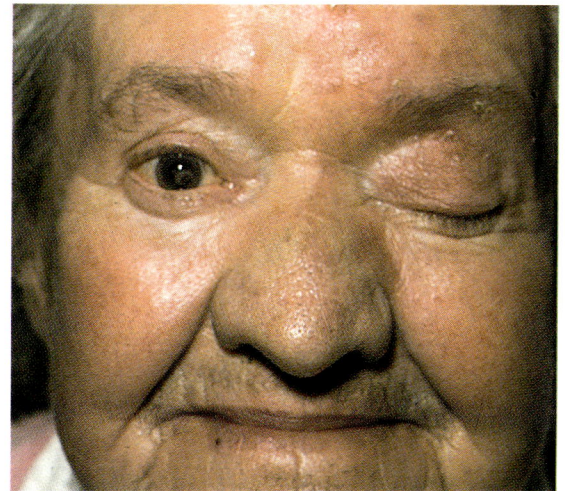

60 Ptosis caused by left oculomotor nerve palsy. Involvement of the cranial nerves supplying extra-ocular muscles occurs in about 10 per cent of cases; it is usually transient and leaves minimal deficit. Residual vesicles are on the left forehead and upper eyelid.

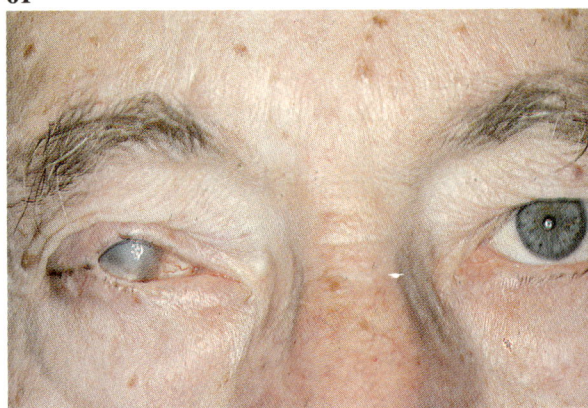

61 Corneal scarring. This is the result of corneal anaesthesia. A protective lateral tarsorrhaphy has been carried out.

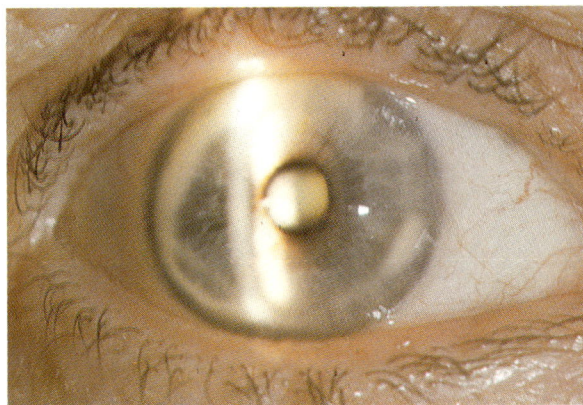

62 Cataract formation, caused by anterior uveitis and secondary glaucoma. A dark area in the iris (at 9 o'clock) represents iris atrophy due to localised vasculitis and is typical of herpes zoster ophthalmicus.

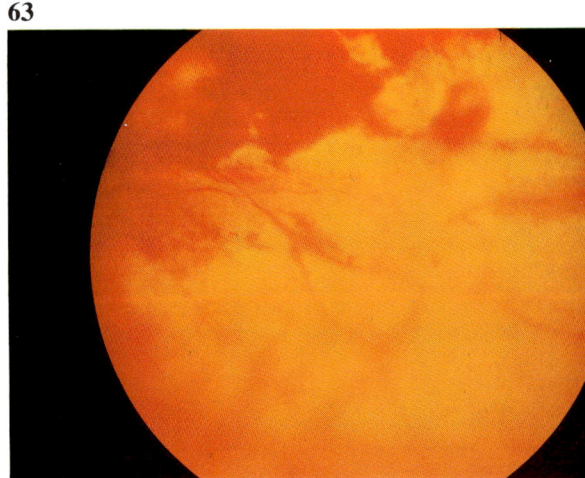

63 Acute retinal necrosis associated with retinal vascular occlusion.

FUNGAL INFECTIONS
Metastatic fungal endophthalmitis

64 Candida albicans retinitis in a drug addict. Inflammatory exudates in the vitreous obscure the fundus view; there are several ill-defined creamy white deposits in the retina.

This may occur when the immune response has been medically suppressed. It is also a hazard of long-term hyperalimentation and of intravenous drug administration by addicts.

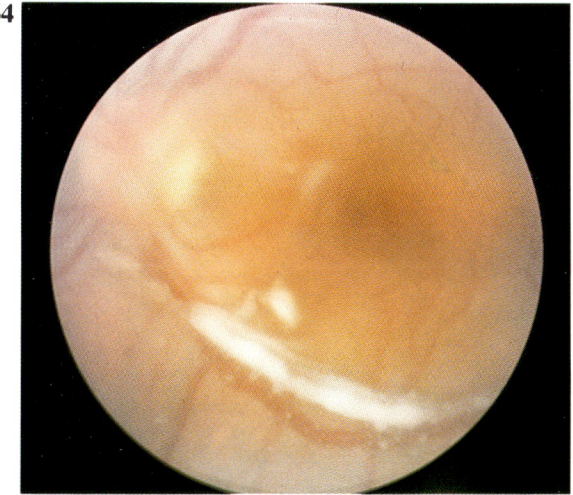

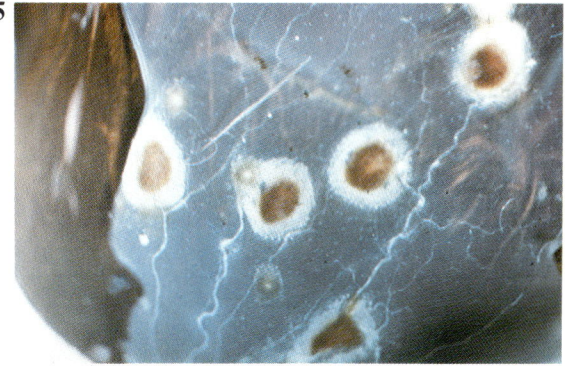

65 Post-mortem specimen. Multiple foci of candida albicans are seen in the retina.

Histoplasmosis

This is a chronic infection of the respiratory system caused by the fungus Histoplasmosis capsulatum; it is endemic in the Ohio and Mississippi river basins. The 'presumed ocular histoplasmosis' syndrome occurs in individuals who have a positive skin reaction to histoplasmosis. It comprises macular haemorrhage and disciform scarring, circumpapillary scarring at the optic disc and scattered atrophic foci in the peripheral fundus ('histo spots'). Although epidemiological studies suggest that histoplasmosis is the cause of the syndrome, similar ocular changes are observed in Europe where histoplasmosis is unknown.

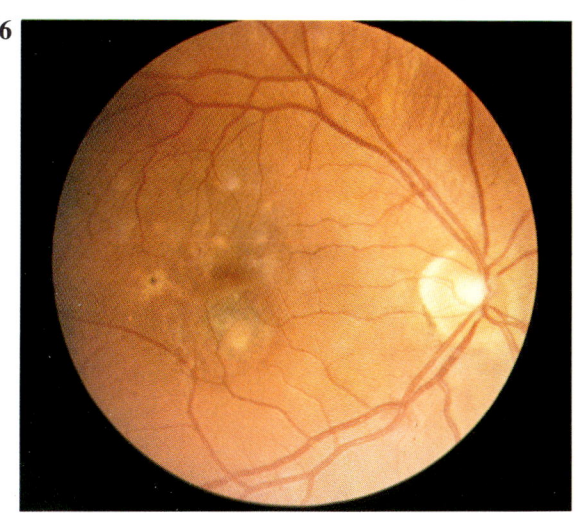

66 Presumed ocular histoplasmosis showing a deep retinal haemorrhage at the macula.

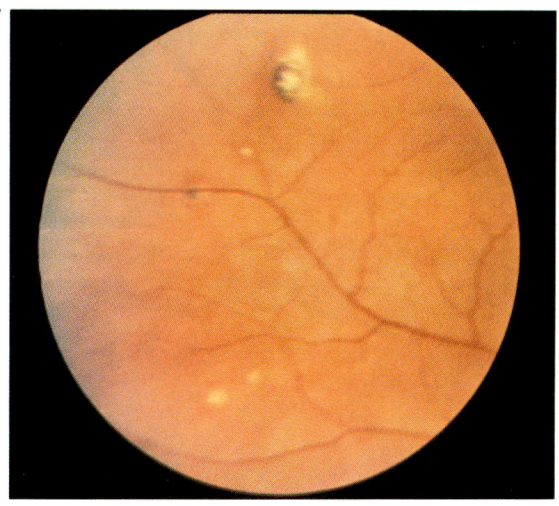

67 'Histo spots' in the peripheral fundus.

PARASITIC INFECTIONS

Toxoplasmosis

This protozoan infection is acquired by contamination from cat faeces or by eating raw or underdone meat. The ingested cysts of Toxoplasmosis gondii release organisms into the gut wall and spread occurs, via the bloodstream and lymphatics, throughout the body. Proliferation of trophozoites causes foci of tissue necrosis surrounded by an intense cellular reaction.

Ocular involvement, in the form of necrotising retinitis, occurs in about 1 per cent of cases with the acquired form of the disease. In congenital toxoplasmosis the eyes are invariably involved; transplacental spread takes place only if the mother is infected during the first trimester of pregnancy.

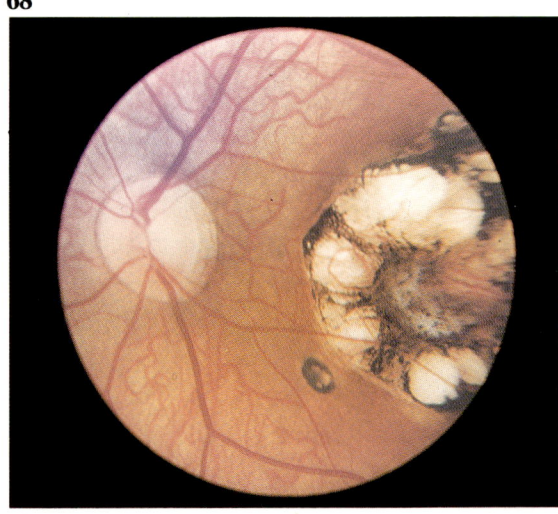

68 Necrotising retinochoroiditis has resulted in a pigmented atrophic scar in the fundus.

Cysticercosis

This is acquired by eating undercooked pork contaminated with eggs of the tapeworm Taenia solium. Embryos released from the eggs penetrate the gut wall and spread via the bloodstream to many organs where the encysted larval stage (cysticerci) develops, notably in subretinal tissue, lens or anterior chamber. Fifty per cent of patients have orbital or intra-ocular involvement.

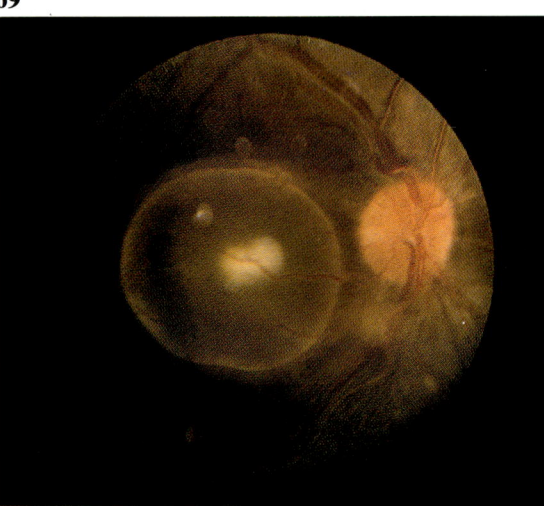

69 Intra-ocular cysticercosis. There is a translucent cyst, containing larvae, visible in the fundus next to the optic disc.

Trichinosis

This nematode infection is contracted by ingestion of meat containing encysted larvae of the roundworm Trichinella spiralis. The larvae penetrate the gut wall and spread via the bloodstream to muscles, to cause widespread myositis, with fever and eosinophilia. Periorbital and facial oedema typically occur.

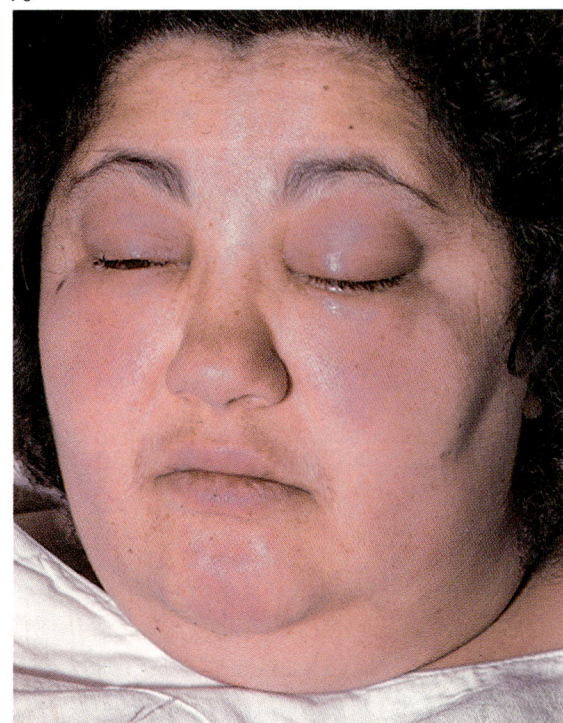

70 Periorbital and facial oedema in trichinosis.

GRANULOMAS

Sarcoidosis

Sarcoidosis is an inflammatory disorder of unknown aetiology affecting nearly all organs of the body. Infection and autoimmune disorders have been implicated, but not proven, as causal agents. The characteristic histological finding is an epithelioid granuloma, similar to that of tuberculosis, but typically without caseation.

The commonest ocular manifestation of sarcoidosis is acute granulomatous uveitis. Other ocular findings include: lacrimal gland infiltration with keratoconjunctivitis sicca (Sjögren's syndrome); proptosis; lagophthalmos caused by recurrent facial nerve palsy; conjunctival infiltration; calcific band keratopathy caused by hypercalcaemia; meningeal infiltration with optic neuritis; retinal periphlebitis with vascular occlusion.

71 Lacrimal gland infiltration in sarcoidosis causes keratoconjunctivitis sicca and is one of the manifestations of Sjögren's syndrome (page 20).

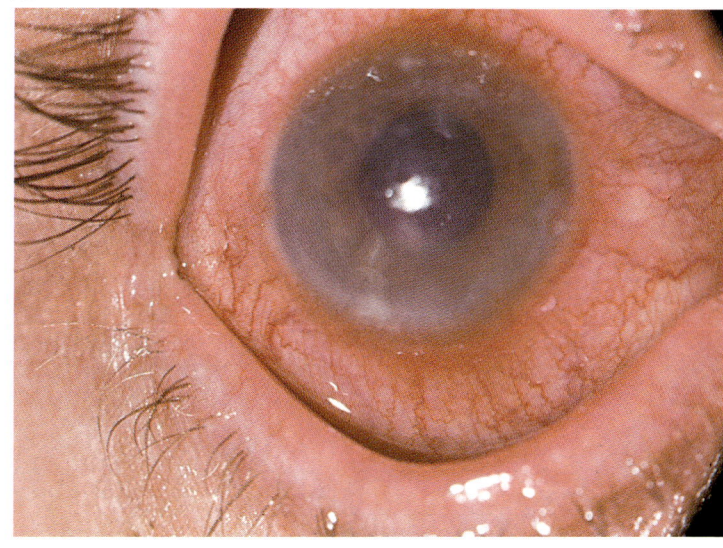

72 Acute granulomatous anterior uveitis (iritis). The injection of ciliary blood-vessels around the limbus of the cornea is typical of iritis. The cornea is hazy due to secondary glaucoma as well as deposits of inflammatory exudate (keratic precipitates) on the inner surface of the cornea.

73 Keratic precipitates on the inner surface of the cornea have a 'mutton fat' appearance, characteristic of sarcoidosis and other granulomatous disorders.

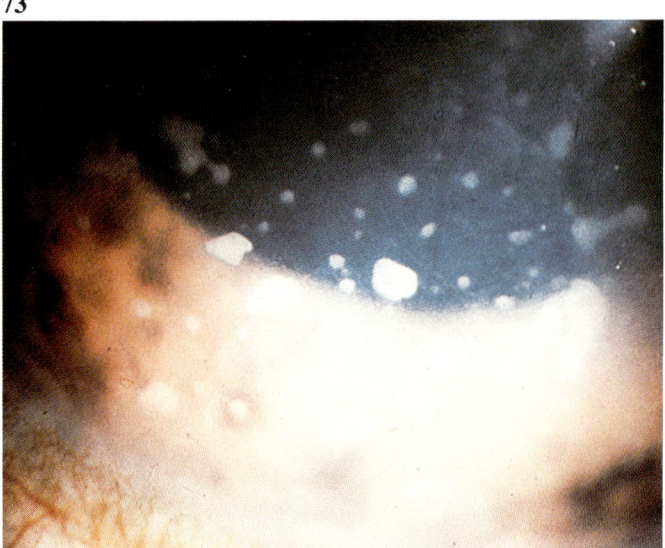

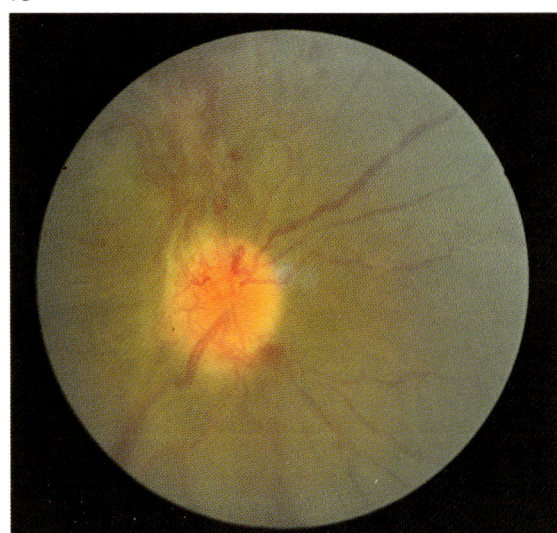

74 Retinal periphlebitis in sarcoidosis is focal in distribution with areas of phlebitis apparently alternating with stretches of unaffected vein.

75 Retinal vein occlusion with retinal haemorrhages secondary to periphlebitis. Retinal ischaemia has stimulated new vessel formation on the optic disc; these new vessels are fragile and prone to haemorrhage.

5: Dermatological disorders

Ocular involvement in dermatological disease includes conditions in which skin and eye lesions are constituents of a clinical pattern; the signs may be topographically related, eg atopic eczema, acne rosacea, herpes zoster ophthalmicus (page 31), or may form part of a systemic syndrome, eg Stevens-Johnson syndrome and the phakomatoses (page 60).

Atopic eczema

In this type of dermatitis, elevated IgE globulin levels are associated with asthma, hay fever, and complications in the anterior structures of the eye.

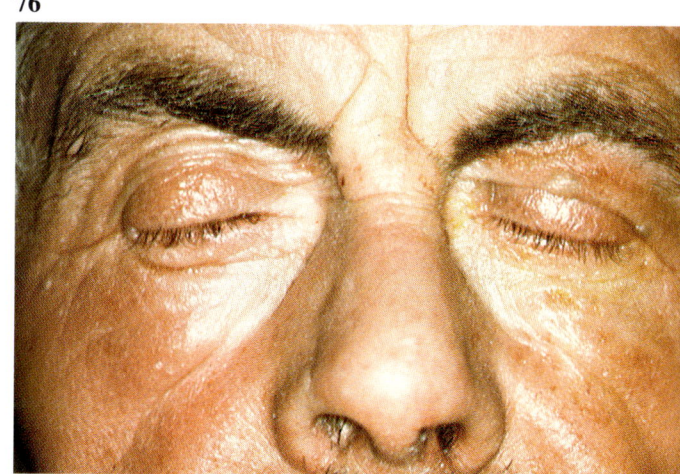

76 Atopic eczema with dry erythema involving the facial skin and eyelids.

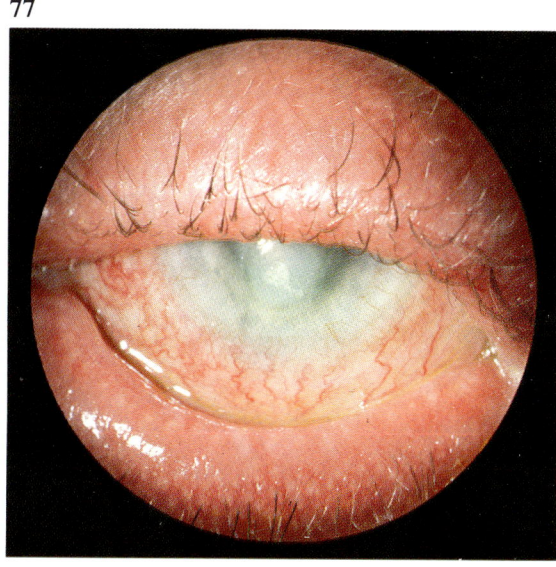

77 Atopic eczema. The skin of the eyelids is thickened and scaling and most of the eyelashes have been lost; conjunctival vessels are dilated and a corneal ulcer (staining yellow-green with fluorescein) affects vision. Vision is further reduced by the presence of a cataract.

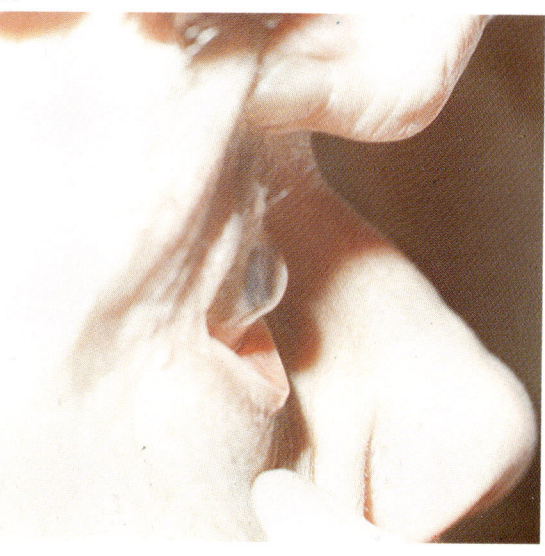

78 Keratoconus. Thinning of the cornea has caused it to bulge forwards. This complication occurs in association with atopic keratoconjunctivitis.

Acne rosacea

This chronic facial dermatitis is characterised by telangiectasia of the skin, facial pustules, diffuse erythema and rhinophyma.

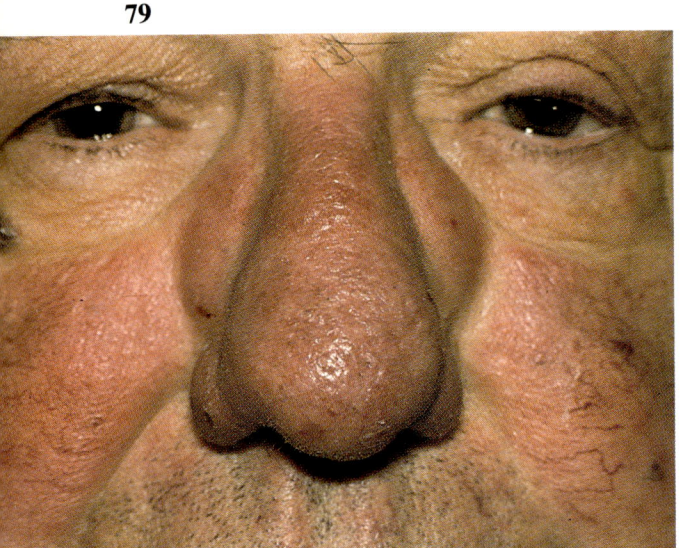

79 Acne rosacea with erythema and telangiectasia of the face and early hypertrophy of the nasal skin (rhinophyma).

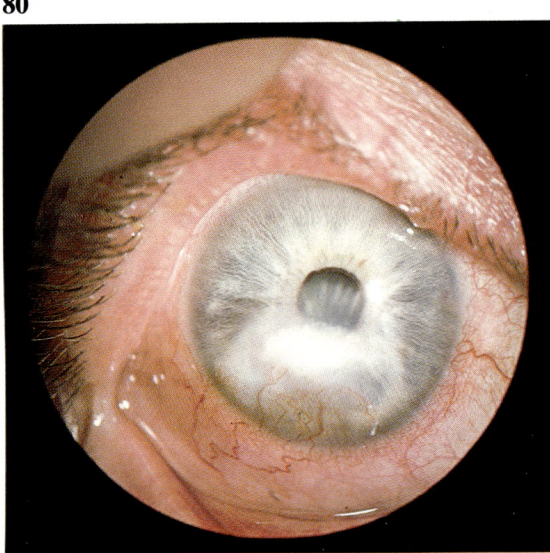

80 Acne rosacea keratoconjunctivitis. Telangiectatic vessels extend from the inflamed conjunctiva on to the cornea and an opaque corneal infiltration obscures vision. The margin of the eyelid is thickened because of chronic blepharitis.

Stevens – Johnson syndrome

This syndrome is a severe form of acute erythema multiforme characterised by extensive immunovasculitis which involves the mucocutaneous tissues of the eyes, mouth and genitalia. This hypersensitivity reaction may be precipitated by a variety of drugs, especially the sulphonomides. It may be caused also by various infections, autoimmune disorders, carcinomas or X-ray therapy.

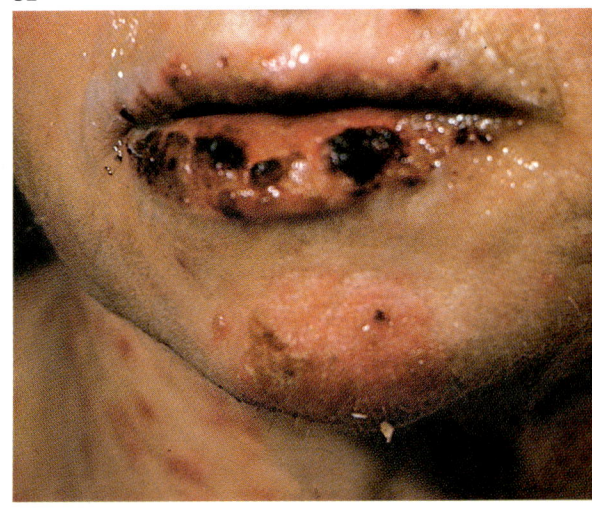

81 Mucocutaneous ulceration in Stevens-Johnson syndrome.

Ocular features include bilateral mucopurulent conjunctivitis which may cause adhesion of the eyelids to the globe (symblepharon). The resultant cicatricial conjunctival fibrosis causes dry eyes, eyelid deformities, corneal exposure and ulceration, uveitis and cataract formation. Spontaneous perforation of the eye may result in panophthalmitis and blindness.

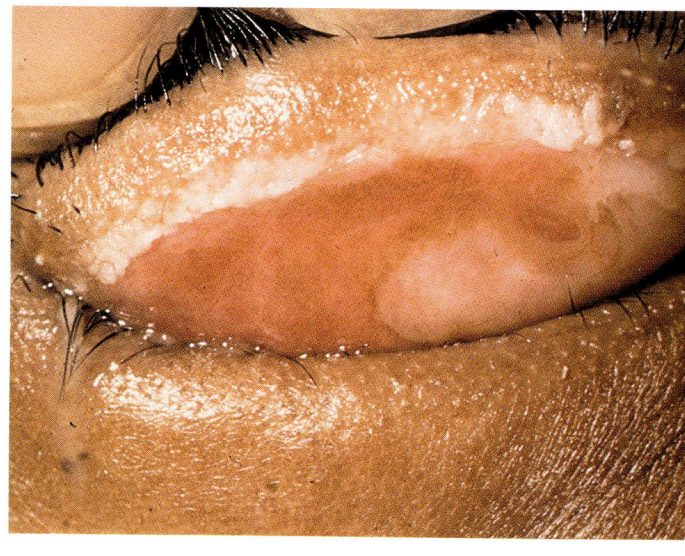

82 Mucopurulent conjunctivitis with early cicatricial conjunctival fibrosis visible inside the everted upper eyelid.

83 Corneal exposure and scarring.

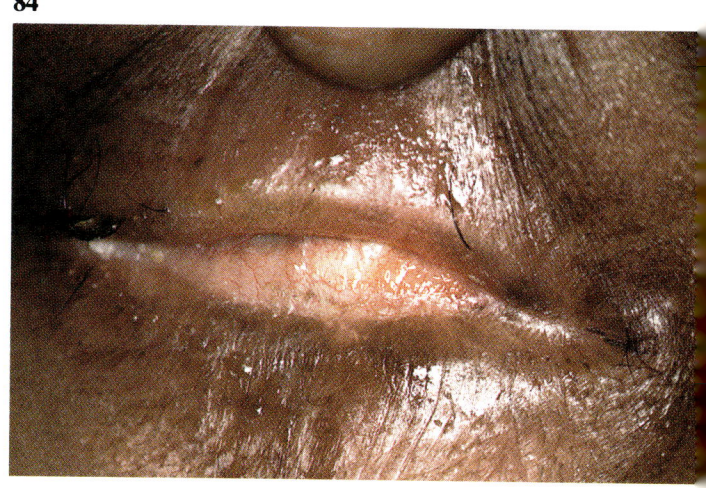

84 Symblepharon preventing opening of the eye.

(Illustrations for figures **83** and **84** by courtesy of Mr M J Roper-Hall.)

6: Endocrine disorders

The most important endocrine disorders which affect the eye are pituitary tumours, Grave's disease and diabetes mellitus. Ocular manifestations of other endocrine disorders are summarised in the following Table.

Endocrine gland	Endocrine disorder	Ocular manifestations
Hypothalamus	Suprasellar tumours	Optic atrophy, papilloedema
Pituitary	Anterior lobe tumours	see page 41
Thyroid	Grave's disease	see page 42
	Myxoedema	Hair loss from eyebrows, periorbital oedema, ptosis, keratoconjunctivitis sicca, cataract, myotonia of extra-ocular muscles
Parathyroids	Hyperparathyroidism	Conjunctival and corneal calcification
	Hypoparathyroidism	Blepharospasm, Chvostek's sign, keratoconjunctivitis, cataract, papilloedema
Pancreas	Diabetes mellitus	see page 44
Adrenals	Pheochromocytoma	Hypertensive retinopathy
	Addison's disease	Pigmentation of eyelids, conjunctiva and uvea
	Cushing's disease	Exophthalmos, hypertensive retinopathy

Pituitary tumours

The close anatomical relationship between the pituitary gland and the optic chiasma accounts for ocular abnormalities associated with anterior lobe tumours: compression of the chiasma leads to optic atrophy and loss of vision. Similarly, the pituitary tumour may invade the adjacent cavernous sinus, leading to damage of the sixth, third and fourth cranial nerves and exophthalmoplegia.

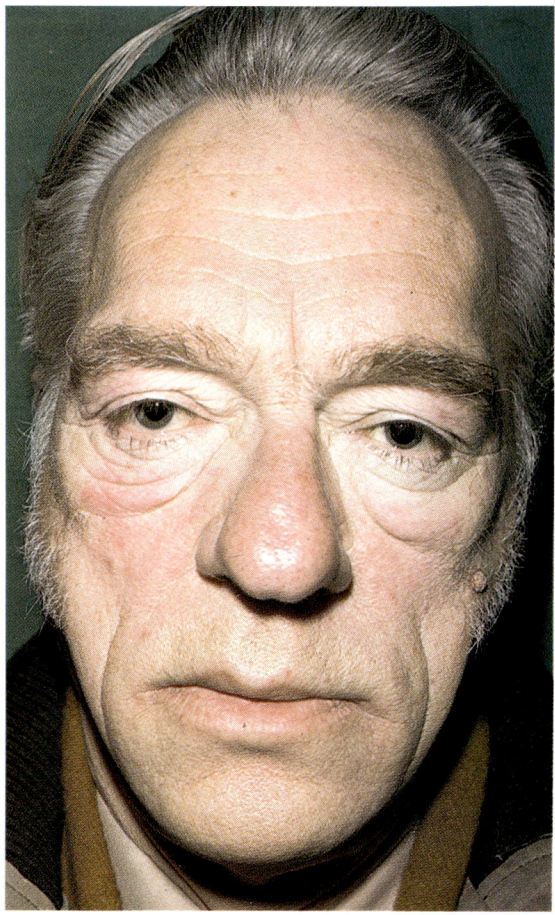

85 Acromegaly. Excess growth hormone secretion by an anterior lobe adenoma has caused overgrowth of the frontal bone and mandible and coarsening of the facial features. Optic atrophy, which may occur, is an indication for neurosurgical intervention.

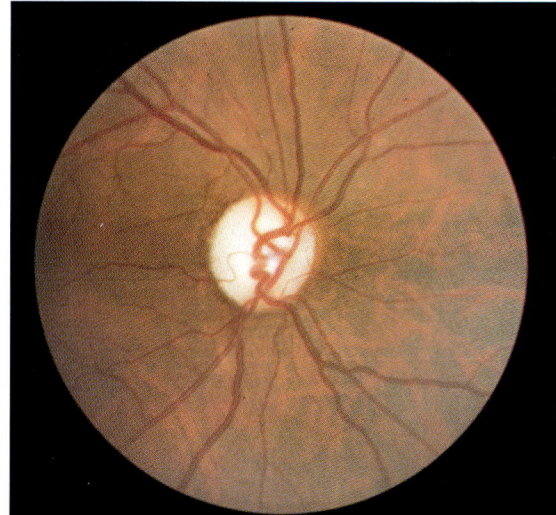

86 Optic atrophy in acromegaly. The flat, pale optic disc has a well-defined margin (primary optic atrophy, page 58). Pituitary tumours typically cause a bitemporal hemianopia.

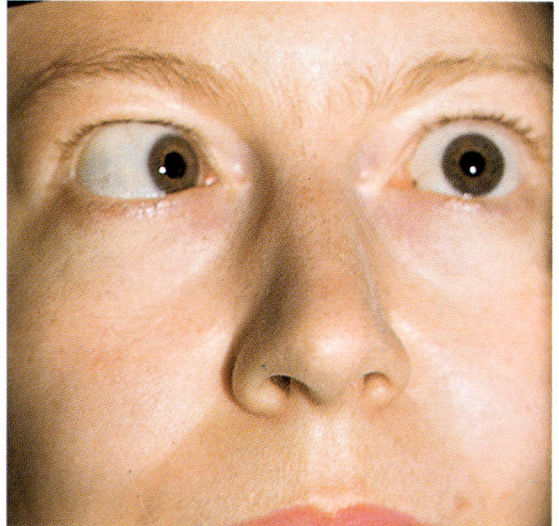

87 Sixth nerve palsy with lack of abduction of the right eye. Invasion of the cavernous sinus by a pituitary tumour usually affects this nerve first because of its more medial position, relative to the third and fourth cranial nerves.

Grave's disease

Grave's disease is an endocrine disorder of uncertain aetiology consisting of a triad of features: hyperthyroidism with diffuse goitre, ophthalmopathy and pretibial myxoedema.

The ocular features of the disease, which vary in severity, have been defined by the American Thyroid Association (based on the classification by Werner) and divided into six classes.

Class	Definition	Clinical features
0	No physical signs or symptoms	Nil
1	Only signs, no symptoms	Lid retraction, lid lag
2	Soft tissue involvement	Oedema of the eyelids, conjunctival injection and oedema, 'gritty' eyes, lacrimation
3	Proptosis	Usually bilateral, not always symmetrical
4	Extra-ocular muscles	Diplopia with upward and lateral gaze first affected
5	Corneal involvement	Exposure keratitis
6	Sight loss (optic nerve involvement)	Papilloedema with secondary optic atrophy

Note: The first letter of each definition forms the mnemonic NO SPECS

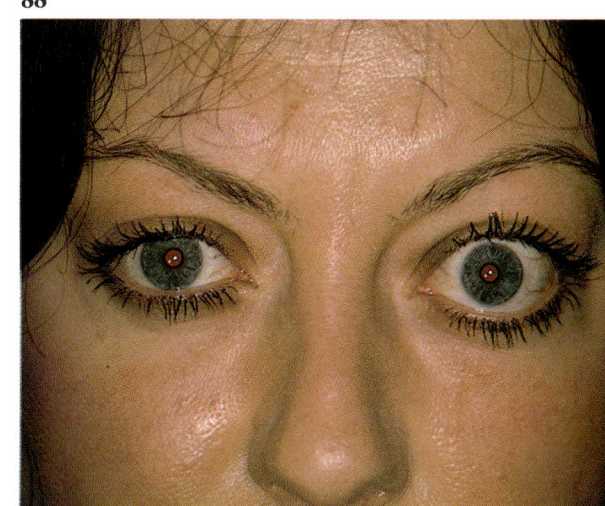

88 Lid retraction with exposure of the sclera above the iris is an early sign of Grave's disease.

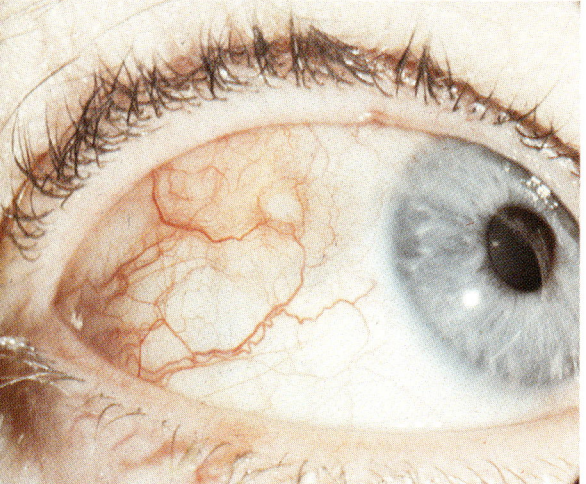

89 Dilatation of the conjunctival vessels typically occurs over the insertion of the lateral rectus muscle.

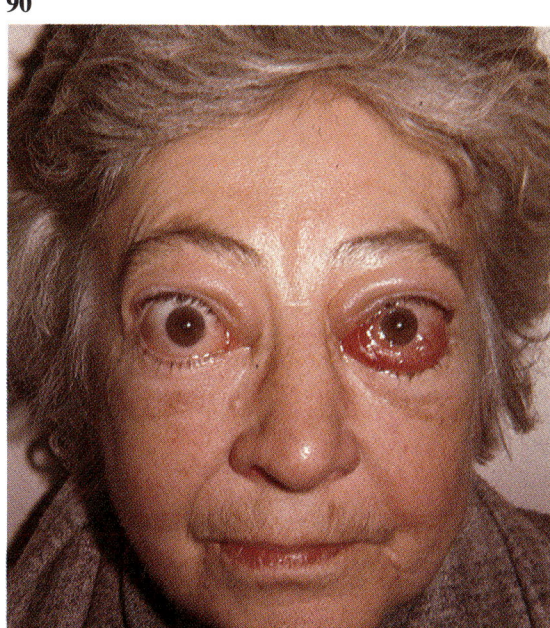

90 Proptosis (exophthalmos) in Grave's disease is usually bilateral but asymmetrical.

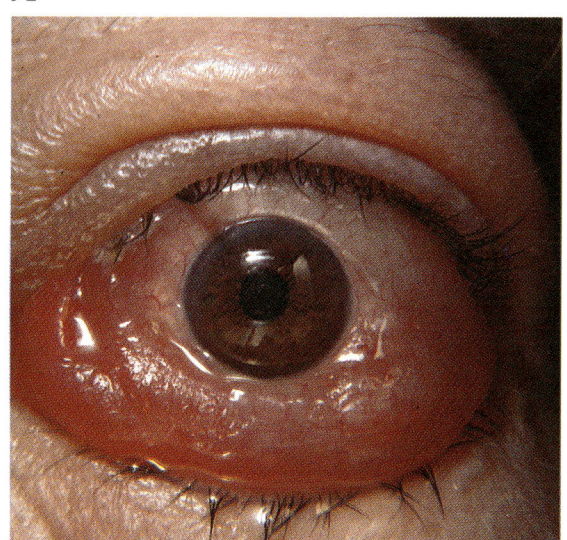

91 (Detail) Proptosis and conjunctival oedema may present acutely and lead to corneal exposure.

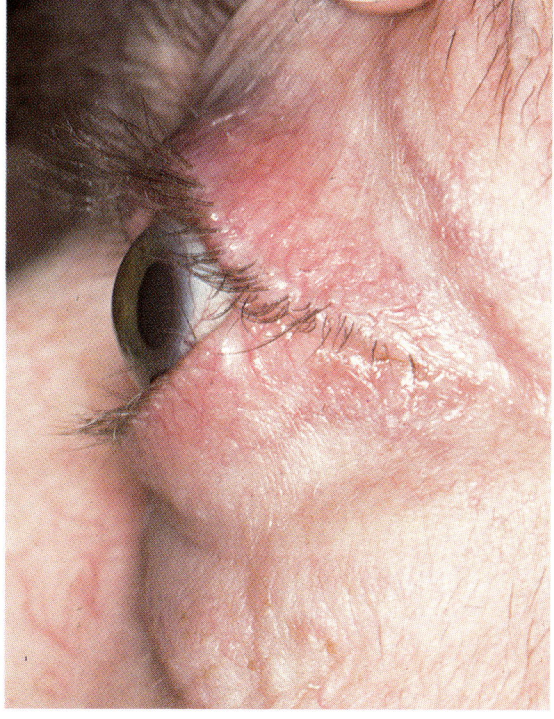

92 Lateral tarsorrhaphy to aid lid closure and prevent corneal exposure.

Diabetes mellitus

Diabetes mellitus has numerous ocular manifestations, listed below. Many aspects of diabetic eye disease affect visual function and diabetic retinopathy is a common cause of blindness.

Eyelids:	xanthelasmata due to hyperlipidaemia (page 12)
Conjunctiva:	microaneurysms, venous dilatation
Extra-ocular muscles:	palsy with diplopia caused by 3rd, 4th or 6th cranial nerve involvement
Orbit:	mucormycosis – a potential complication of severe diabetic acidosis
Iris:	neovascularisation of the anterior surface (rubeosis iridis)
Glaucoma:	neovascular glaucoma, chronic open angle glaucoma
Pupil:	poor dilatation caused by rubeosis iridis, Argyll-Robertson pupil
Lens:	cataract, refractive errors
Vitreous body:	vitreous haemorrhage, asteroid hyalosis
Retina:	diabetic retinopathy, retinal vein occlusion (page 49), lipaemia retinalis (page 12).
Optic nerve:	ischaemic papillitis, optic atrophy (page 58)

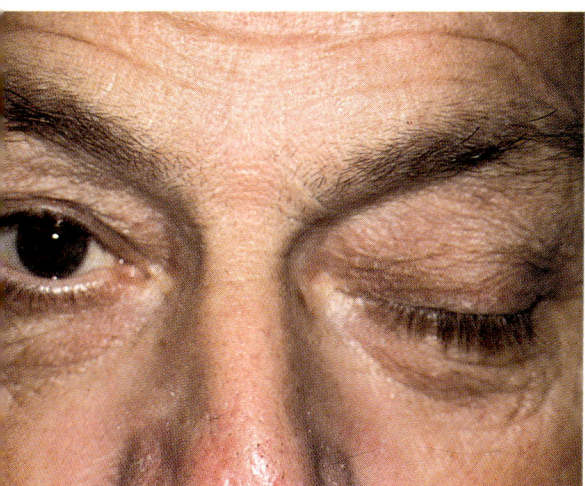

93 Ptosis caused by oculomotor nerve palsy. Cranial nerve function usually recovers within three months. Sparing of the pupil distinguishes diabetic third nerve palsy from that caused by mechanical factors such as aneurysm or neoplasm.

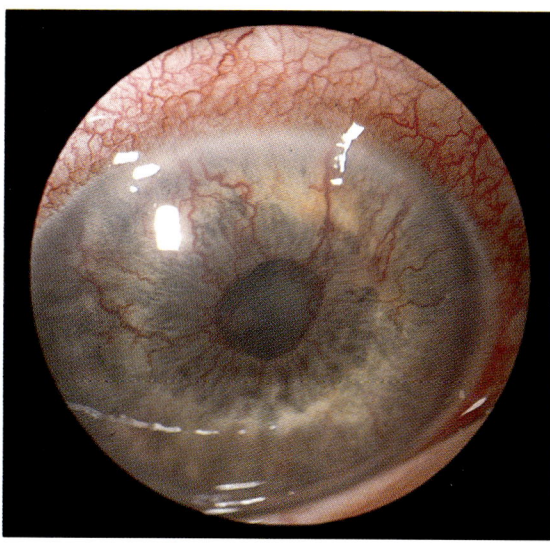

94 Rubeosis iridis. New vessels develop on the anterior surface of the iris in response to severe ocular ischaemia. Consequent obstruction of aqueous drainage results in neovascular glaucoma.

Rubeosis iridis may also occur secondary to central retinal vein occlusion, intraocular tumours, long-standing retinal detachments and carotid stenosis.

95 Senile cataract. This occurs at a younger age in diabetics than in other patients.

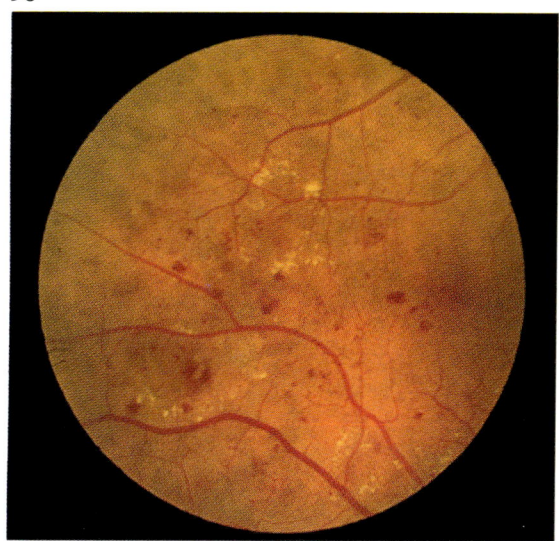

96 Background diabetic retinopathy with microaneurysms (dots), retinal haemorrhages (blots) and yellow hard exudates; vision may not be affected in the early stages.

97 Fluorescein angiogram in diabetic retinopathy showing dark ischaemic areas of 'capillary dropout' (C), microaneurysms (M) and leakage (L) from new vessels on the optic disc.

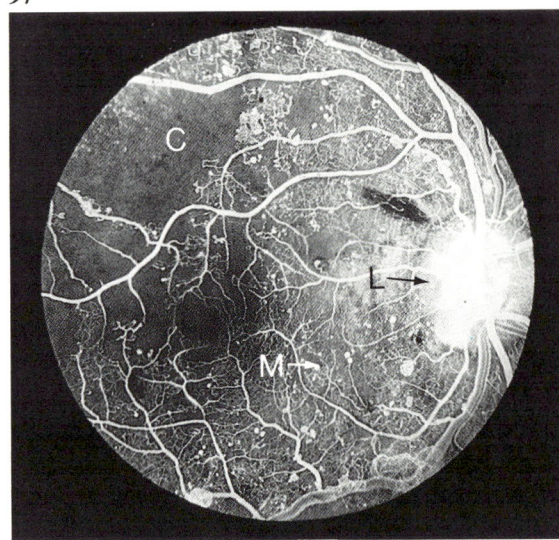

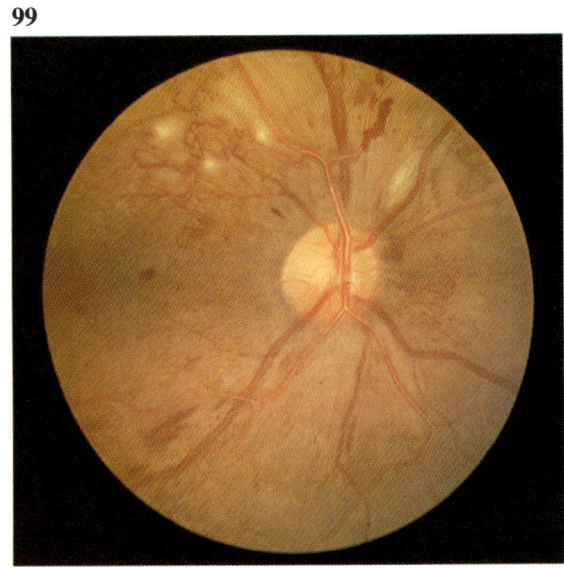

98 Diabetic maculopathy. Yellow hard exudates form a circinate pattern in the macula causing loss of central vision.

99 Pre-proliferative diabetic retinopathy. 'Cotton-wool spots' and venous beading indicate progression of the retinopathy and precede new vessel formation.

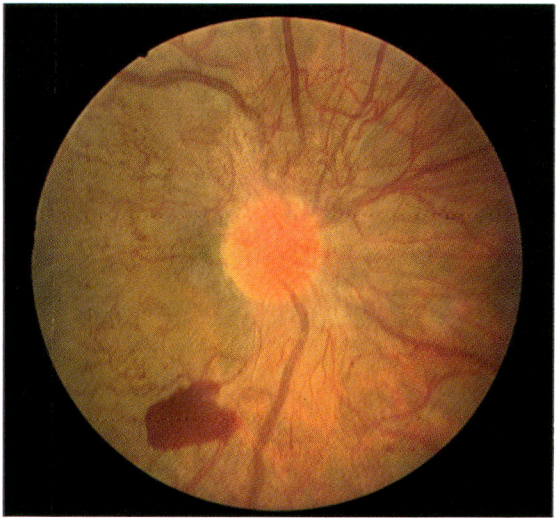

100 Proliferative retinopathy. Retinal ischaemia leads to formation of new vessels on the optic disc.

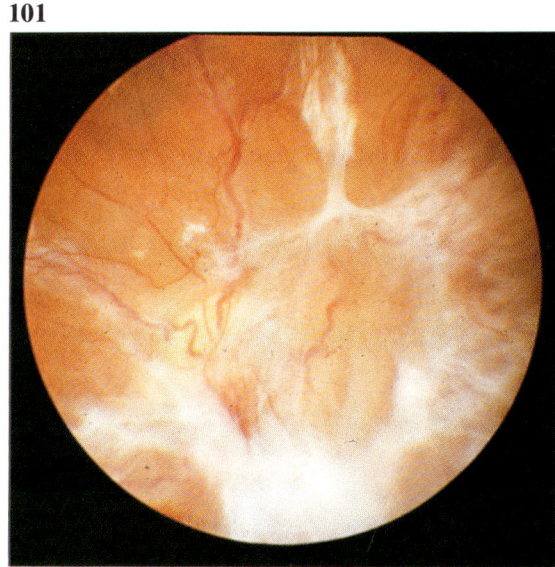

101 Traction retinal detachment caused by fibrous proliferation in advanced diabetic retinopathy.

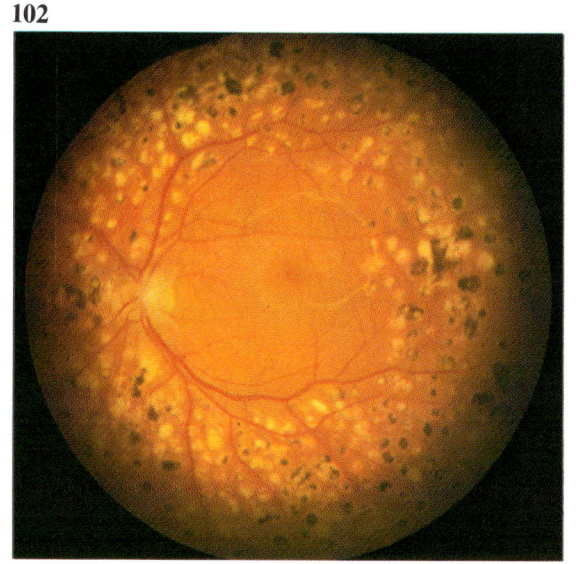

102 Argon laser panphotocoagulation for treatment of proliferative diabetic retinopathy has resulted in numerous pigmented scars in the peripheral retina. Dark adaptation may be affected.

7: Cardiovascular and pulmonary disorders

The blood vessels of the optic fundus are clearly visible with the ophthalmoscope. Thus many pathological features associated with systemic disorders, such as hypertension, cyanotic congenital heart disease and respiratory insufficiency, can be observed directly. Similarly, retinal vascular accidents, for example arterial or venous occlusion, may reflect systemic disorders; emboli originating from the heart or large blood-vessels, or from neoplasms, frequently lodge in the eye.

CARDIOVASCULAR DISORDERS

Systemic hypertension

Changes in the retinal vessels reflect the rate of progression and severity of systemic hypertension. Mild hypertension causes irregularities in arteriolar calibre, sinusoidal tortuosity of the retinal arterioles and changes at arteriovenous crossings. Accelerated hypertension is associated with generalised arteriolar narrowing and various degrees of retinal ischaemia (manifested as 'cotton-wool spots', haemorrhages, retinal oedema) and papilloedema.

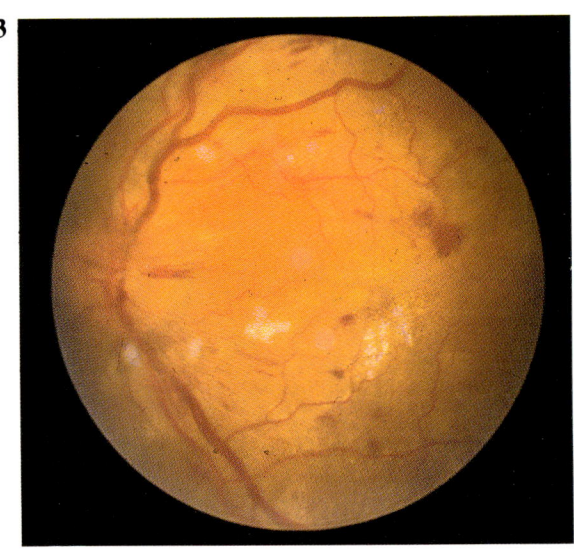

103 Accelerated hypertension. The retinal arterioles are attenuated and irregular in outline; hard exudates surround the macula in a radiating pattern ('macular star'); soft exudates ('cotton-wool spots') indicate the presence of nerve fibre layer infarcts due to ischaemia; papilloedema reflects the severity of the hypertension.

Retinal artery occlusion

This ocular abnormality is associated with a wide variety of systemic disorders. It may occur secondary to atherosclerosis, arteriosclerosis, hypertension, hyperlipidaemia (page 12) or vasculitis (page 24); it can be brought about by decreased blood flow to the retina, as in carotid stenosis, or it may be caused by emboli from the heart or large vessels.

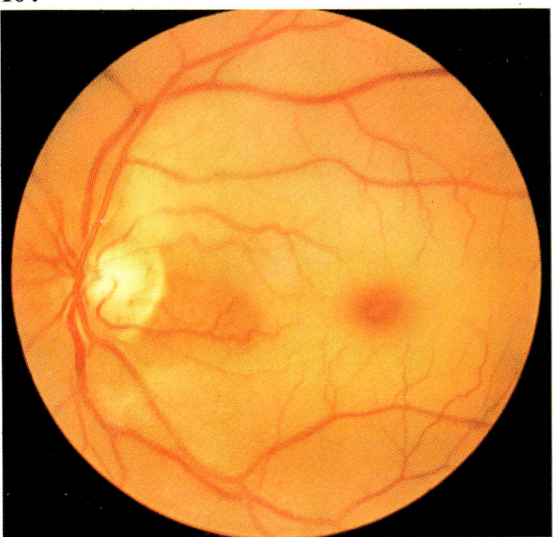

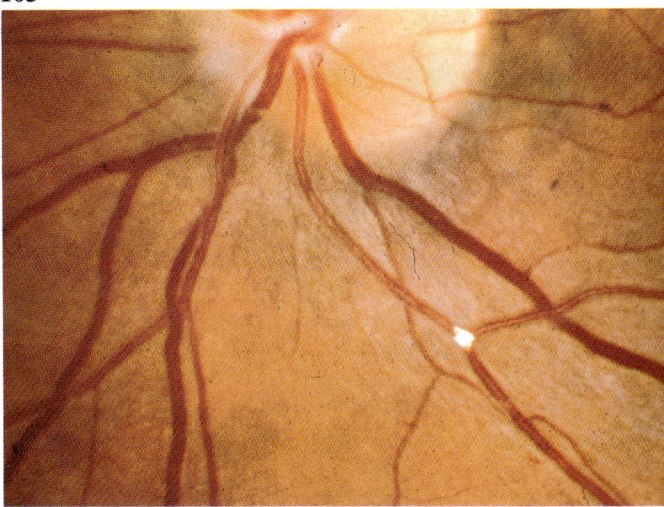

104 Central retinal artery occlusion. The retinal arterioles are attenuated and the retina pale and oedematous, except for the fovea (supplied by the underlying choroidal circulation) which shows as a 'cherry-red spot'; the optic disc is pale and swollen.

105 Retinal arterial embolism. There is a shiny yellow lipid embolus lodged in the bifurcation of a retinal arteriole. It originated from an atheromatous plaque in the carotid artery. The presenting symptom was amaurosis fugax.

The heart is another possible source of retinal emboli, which can be calcific, myxomatous, or septic in nature.

Retinal vein occlusion

The systemic disorders associated with retinal vein occlusion are similar to those of retinal artery occlusion; in addition retinal vein occlusion may be found in association with diabetes mellitus (page 44) and hyperviscosity of the blood (page 54).

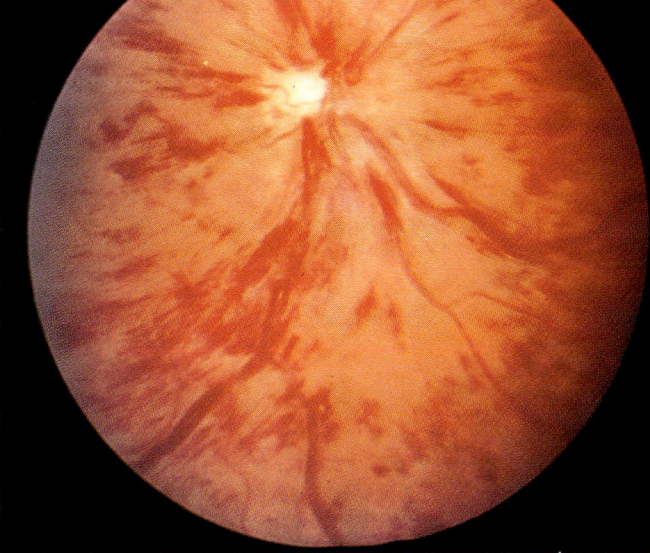

106 Central retinal vein occlusion. There are multiple haemorrhages scattered over the retina, partially obscuring the dilated retinal veins; the optic disc is swollen and congested; associated severe retinal ischaemia may lead to the development of rubeosis iridis (page 45).

Cyanotic congenital heart disease

The ocular features of this group of disorders are caused by hypoxia and central cyanosis.

107

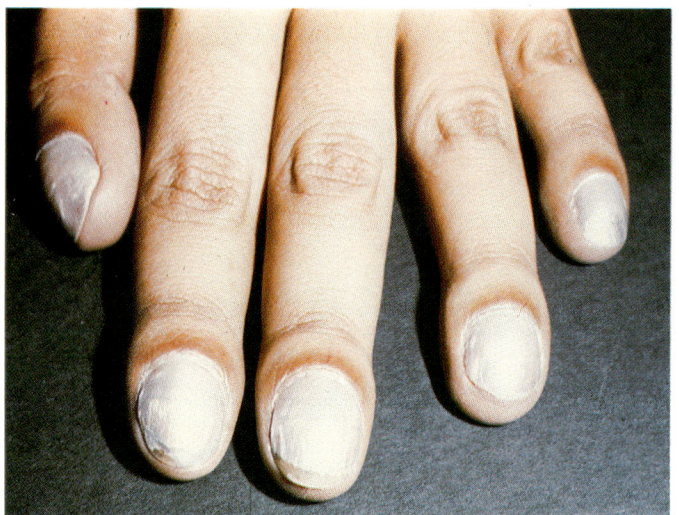

108

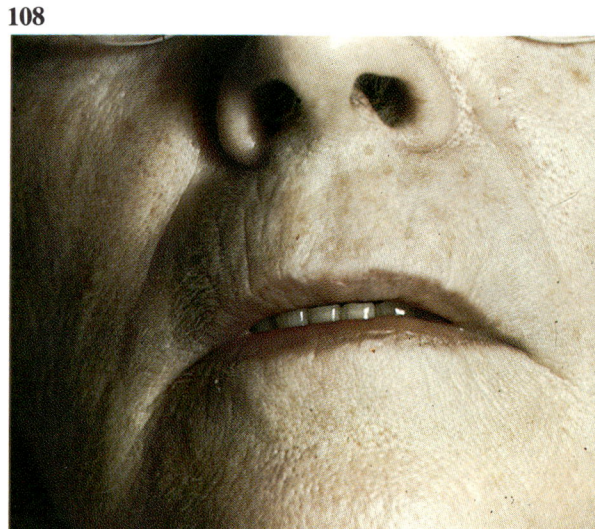

107 Clubbing of the fingers is a characteristic of cyanotic congenital heart disease.

108 Discoloration of the lips in central cyanosis.

109

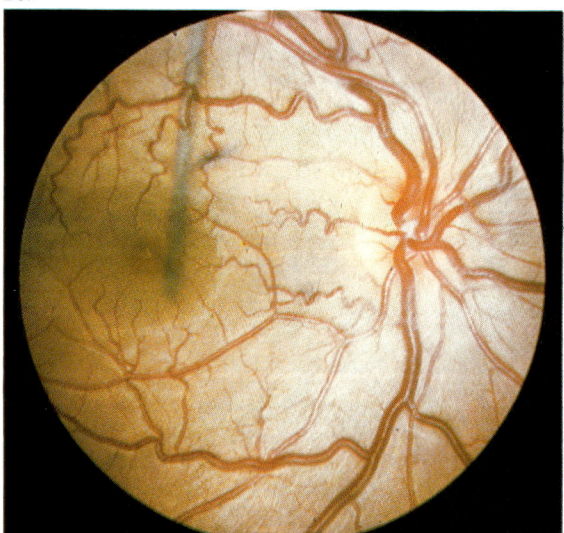

PULMONARY DISORDERS
Respiratory insufficiency

Papilloedema occurs in cases of severe respiratory insufficiency due to hypercapnia which increases cerebral and retinal blood flow.

110

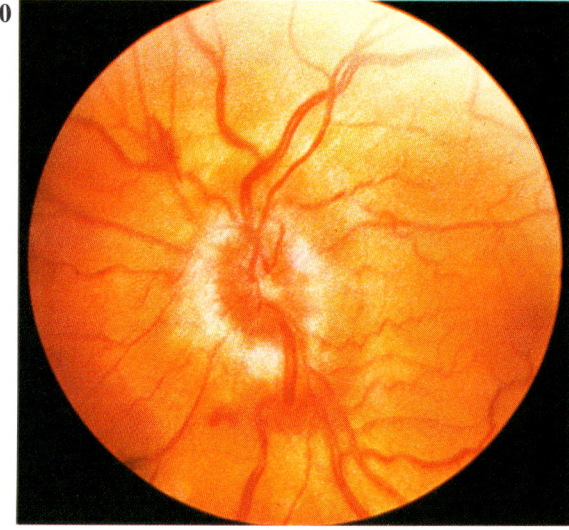

109 Retinal cyanosis. The retina has a purple hue and the veins are engorged because of secondary polycythaemia. (The dark vertical line is a macular fixation target superimposed on the camera lens.)

110 Papilloedema in respiratory insufficiency. The swollen optic disc has an ill-defined margin and the retinal veins are dilated and tortuous. This ocular abnormality may also occur in other systemic disorders (page 59).

Bronchial carcinoma

Direct and/or metastatic spread from the primary tumour may affect the eye.

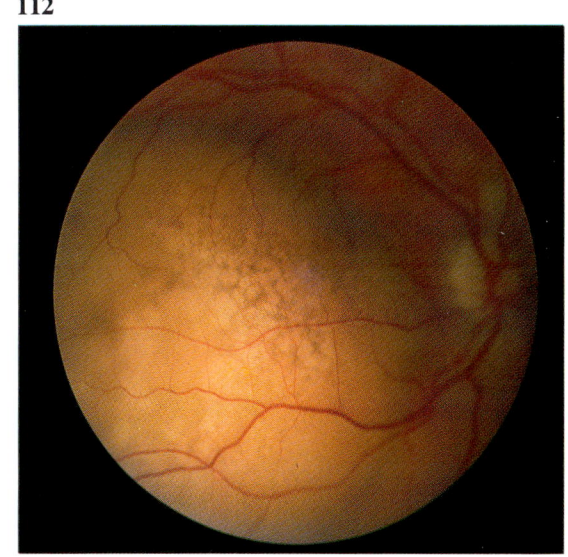

111 Horner's syndrome. The right eye is enophthalmic with ptosis and miosis; the patient had anhidrosis on this side of the face.

Horner's syndrome may be caused by infiltration of the cervical sympathetic ganglia by bronchial carcinoma in the apex of the lung; this combination is known as Pancoast's syndrome.

112 Choroidal metastasis. There is a large pale raised mass in the fundus underlying the retinal vessels. The optic disc lies in a different plane and is out of focus.

Bronchial carcinoma frequently metastasises to the fundus, as do other tumours such as carcinoma of the breast.

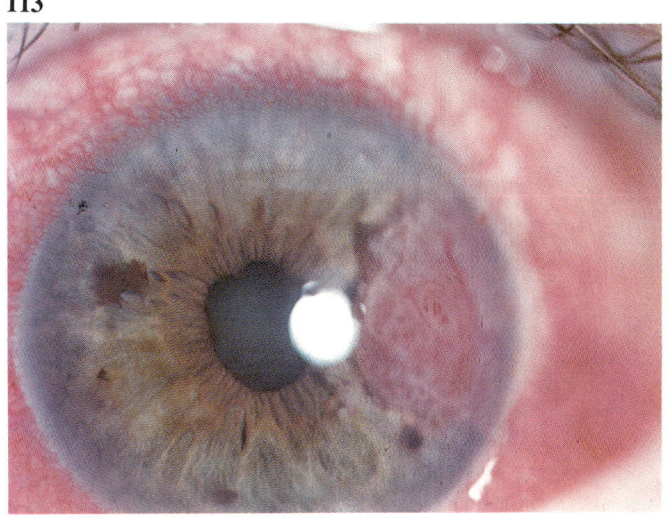

113 Iris metastasis. In this patient with carcinoma of the bronchus there is a metastasis in the iris; it forms a fleshy pink lump in the anterior chamber of the eye and can be seen through the cornea.

8: Renal disorders

Renal disorders are associated with a wide range of ocular abnormalities. With a few exceptions, however, these ocular abnormalities are non-specific and present as secondary phenomena, related to a clinical spectrum of systemic disorders which include the renal system. For example, renal failure is associated with hypertension and some ocular features are common to both conditions. Similarly, the manifestations of inherited renal disease frequently involve abnormalities of other systems, as well as of the eye. In addition, disturbances occur in the eye arising from complications of renal transplant procedures.

The ocular features of renal disorders can be summarised as follows:

Renal failure associated with:
— hypertension – hypertensive retinopathy (page 48) and encephalopathy with cranial nerve palsies

— chronic hypocalcaemia – cataracts

— chronic hyperphosphataemia – metastatic calcification of conjunctiva and cornea

— uric acid retention – gouty iritis (page 23)

Inherited renal disorders
— metabolic abnormalities – Wilson's disease (page 9), homocystinuria (page 10), galactosaemia (page 11)

— phakomatoses – von Hippel-Lindau syndrome (page 64)

Complications of renal transplant
— immunosuppressive therapy – opportunistic infections including herpes simplex dendritic ulcer, cytomegalovirus retinitis; cataract (systemic steroids)

114

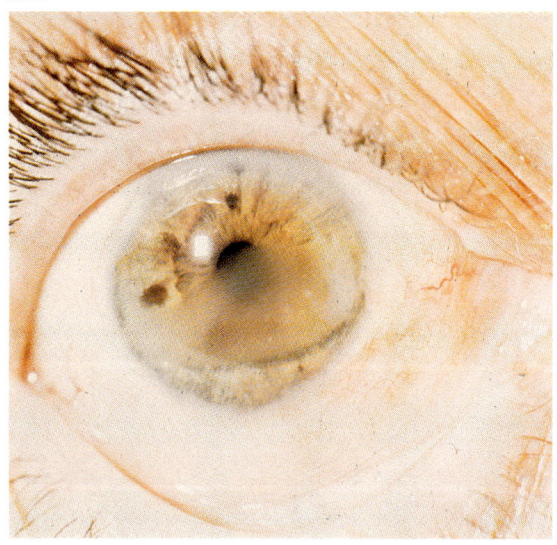

114 Corneal calcification in chronic renal failure.

115

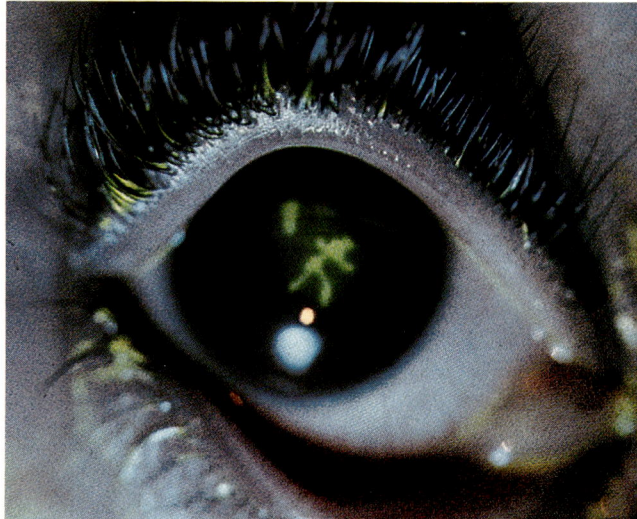

115 Dendritic ulcer of the cornea caused by herpes simplex virus; staining of the ulcer with fluorescein reveals its branching structure. The patient was receiving immunosuppressive therapy.

9: Haemopoetic and lymphoreticular disorders

Abnormalities in the number and structure of red blood cells, changes in blood viscosity, and disorders of the lymphoreticular system are associated with numerous ocular manifestations, many of which affect vision.

Anaemia

Anaemia, from whatever cause, is typically associated with abnormalities of the ocular fundus, although ophthalmological signs usually only become apparent when the concentration of red blood cells is reduced to about 50 per cent of normal. Retinal haemorrhages are the commonest manifestation, but subconjunctival haemorrhages may occur.

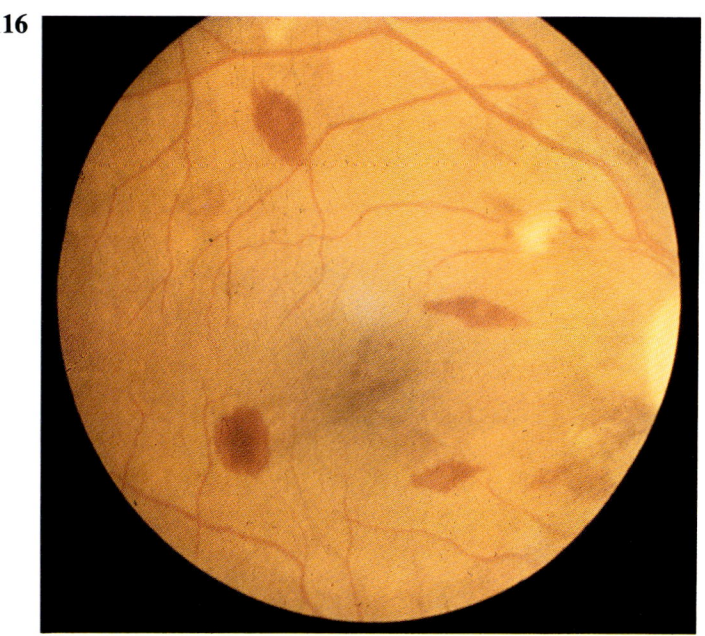

116 Anaemia. The fundus is pale and the retinal arterioles and venules appear similar in colour; there are scattered soft exudates ('cotton-wool spots') and deep retinal haemorrhages, typically with a white centre and dark periphery (Roth spots).

Other fundoscopic abnormalities associated with anaemia include: hard exudates with 'macular star' formation (severe, chronic anaemia); preretinal or subhyaloid haemorrhages which may rupture into the vitreous; exudative retinal detachment and optic atrophy (pernicious anaemia).

Polycythaemia

An excess of circulating red blood cells, with an associated increase in blood viscosity, results in venous engorgement of the eye. Thus the iris may assume a red-brown hue and the fundus appear cyanotic. The engorged retinal veins are prone to occlusion and retinal haemorrhage is common; papilloedema may also occur (page 59). Amaurosis fugax, caused by involvement of the vertebrobasilar system, may be a presenting symptom. Intra-cranial thrombosis and haemorrhage may result in exophthalmoplegia and diplopia.

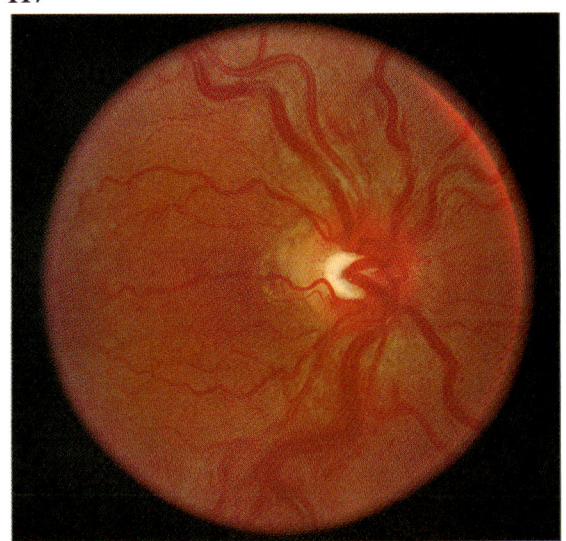

117 The fundus in polycythaemia with engorged and tortuous vessels.

Other causes of blood hyperviscosity, such as macroglobulinaemia and paraproteinaemia, may produce a similar appearance.

Sickle cell disease

Sickle cell disease refers to those genetically determined haemoglobinopathies in which a single amino acid substitution results in an abnormal haemoglobin molecule which causes red blood cells to take on a 'sickle' shape when exposed to an environment of decreased oxygenation. The disease has a high prevalence among ethnic groups originating from Africa, the Mediterranean, the Middle East, and the Indian subcontinent. Individuals with haemoglobin SC, SS and S-thalassaemia are particularly likely to show ocular signs.

Ocular complications are the result of secondary vascular changes and/or occlusion by the sickle-shaped cells. The conjunctival vessels undergo 'comma-shaped' dilatation with saccular aneurysm formation. A typical retinopathy occurs and is divided into nonproliferative and proliferative stages.

Non-proliferative retinopathy consists of retinal haemorrhages ('salmon patches') which may evolve into pigmented retinal scars ('black sunbursts'). Whitening of the peripheral retina and retinal vascular tortuosity also occur.

Proliferative retinopathy is characterised by peripheral retinal vascular occlusion, arteriovenous anastomoses, and the development of retinal neovascularisation ('sea fans') at the junction of the perfused and non-perfused retina. Progressive neovascularisation leads to recurrent vitreous haemorrhage and secondary traction detachment of the retina.

Angioid streaks (page 16) may present as an additional retinal abnormality at any stage of the development of the retinopathy.

118 Sickle cell retinopathy with a pale pink retinal haemorrhage ('salmon patch') and tortuous retinal vessels.

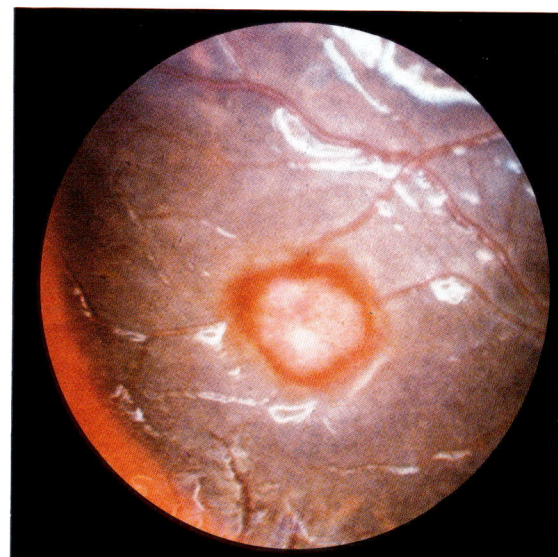

119 Sickle cell retinopathy. Peripheral neovascularisation forms a typical 'sea fan' pattern.

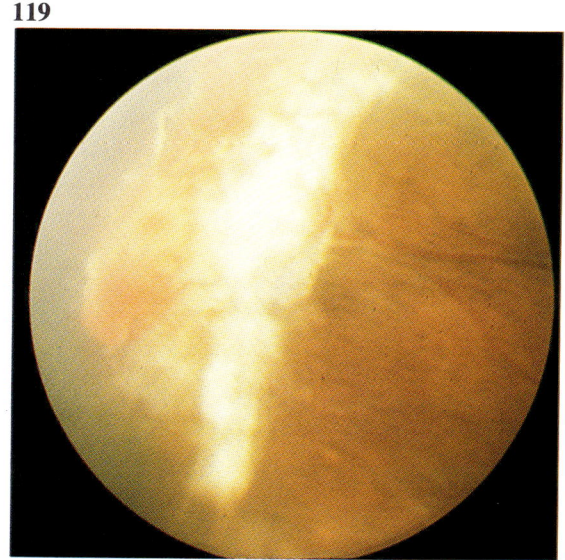

120 Fluorescein angiogram. The peripheral retina is dark and under-perfused due to vascular occlusion; the adjacent 'sea fan' is formed by an arcade of neovascularisation.

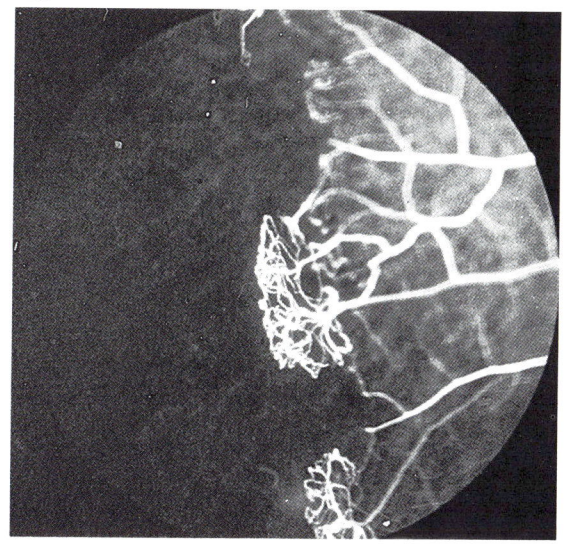

Lymphoreticular neoplasms

Malignant tumours of the lymphoreticular system include the leukaemias, Hodgkin's disease and other lymphomas.

Ophthalmic abnormalities occur secondary to infiltration of tissues, haemorrhage or infection. They include the following features:

Orbit:	proptosis
Eyelids:	ptosis caused by cranial nerve involvement
Lacrimal system:	dacrocystitis with obstruction of lacrimal drainage, lacrimal gland infiltration causing Sjögren's syndrome (page 20)
Extra-ocular muscles:	ophthalmoplegia with diplopia
Conjunctiva:	thickening due to infiltration, subconjunctival haemorrhage
Iris:	infiltration and hyperaemia, hypopyon, spontaneous haemorrhage with hyphaema
Fundus:	leukaemic deposits, perivascular infiltrates, papilloedema, changes due to associated anaemia (page 53)

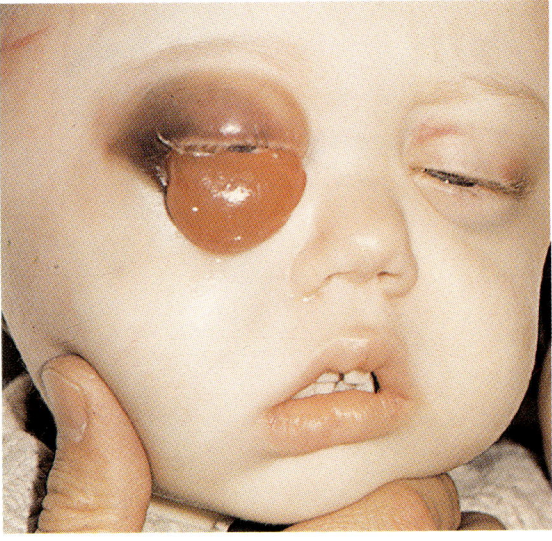

121 Acute leukaemia with proptosis secondary to orbital infiltration and haemorrhage. (Illustration by courtesy of the late Dr W H P Cant.)

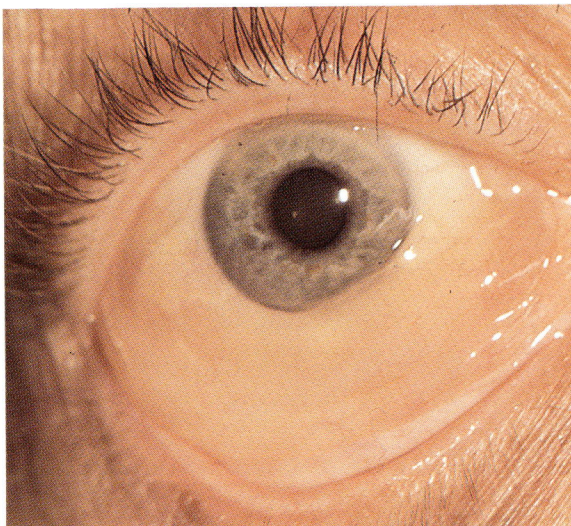

122 Hodgkin's disease. The conjunctival infiltrate has a smooth fleshy appearance and is typically situated in the inferior fornix.

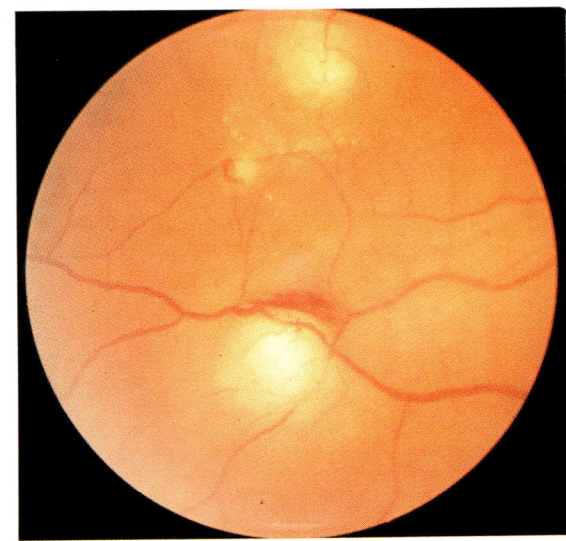

123 Leukaemic retinal infiltrates with an associated retinal haemorrhage caused by secondary anaemia.

10: Gastrointestinal and hepatobiliary disorders

Gastrointestinal and hepatobiliary disorders are associated with a wide variety of ocular abnormalities. With a few exceptions, these ocular abnormalities are non-specific and generally occur secondary to the associated involvement of other systems.

The ocular manifestations of gastrointestinal and hepatobiliary disorders can be classified and summarised as follows:

Inflammatory bowel disease
— Crohn's disease, ulcerative colitis – episcleritis and anterior uveitis

Malabsorption syndrome
— Vitamin deficiencies – see ocular features of anaemia (page 53)
— dark adaptation, xerophthalmia and Bitot spots (Vitamin A deficiency)
— Abetalipoproteinaemia – retinitis pigmentosa (page 14)

Peptic and neoplastic bowel disorders
— Chronic haemorrhage – see ocular features of anaemia (page 53)
— Acute severe haemorrhage – optic neuritis and atrophy (page 58)

Vascular bowel anomalies
— Rendu-Osler-Weber syndrome (page 18)

Hepatobiliary disease
— Bile obstruction – jaundice
— Hyperlipidaemia (page 12)
— Gastrointestinal haemorrhage (see above)
— Wilson's disease (page 9)

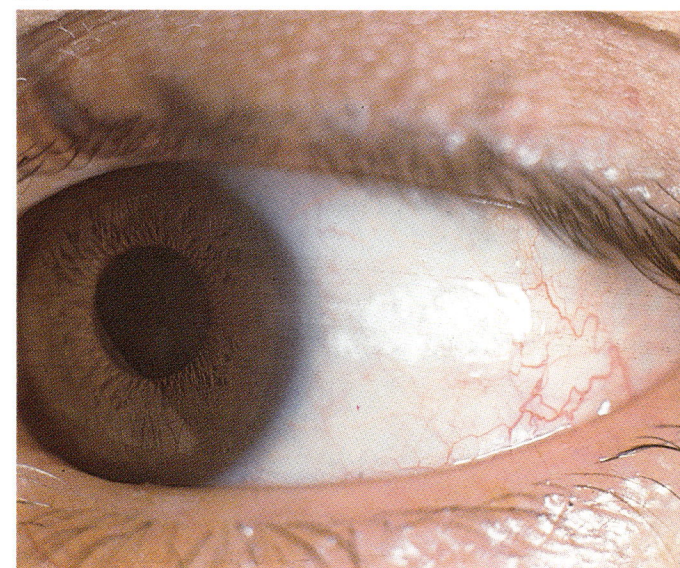

124 Bitot spot in Vitamin A deficiency. A localised area of xerosis forms a small foamy white plaque on the lateral conjunctiva.

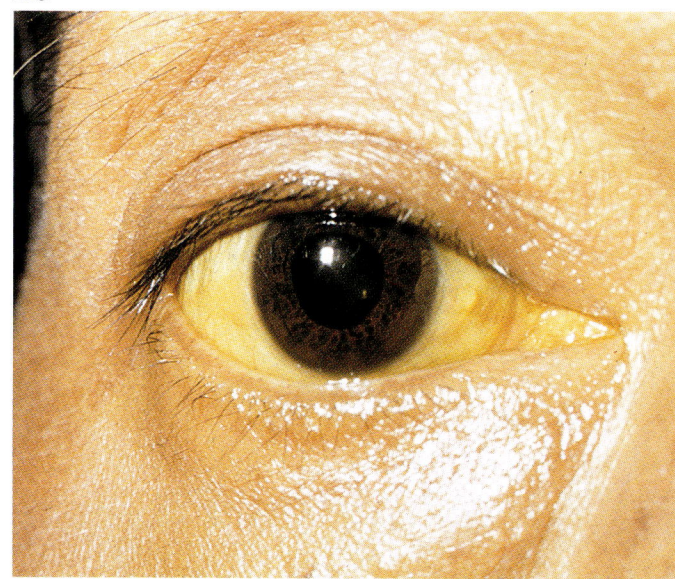

125 Jaundice is a common manifestation of hepatobiliary disease; the conjunctiva and sclera are stained yellow by bile pigments.

11: Neurological and muscle disorders

Systemic and intracranial disorders may affect the optic nerve, causing changes in the appearance of the optic disc on fundoscopy (papillitis, optic atrophy, papilloedema). Exophthalmoplegia with diplopia due to involvement of the third, fourth or sixth cranial nerves are similarly caused by a wide range of systemic conditions, referred to in other sections. The phakomatoses are congenital disorders of ectodermal tissues characterised by ocular, neurological and dermatological hamartomas. The ocular abnormalities associated with the muscle disorders myasthenia gravis and myotonic dystrophy may assist in the diagnosis of these conditons.

OPTIC NERVE AND OPTIC DISC ABNORMALITIES

Optic neuritis

The optic nerve may be affected in any part of its course by inflammatory, degenerative or demyelinating disease; severe systemic haemorrhage occasionally may cause optic neuritis.

Involvement of the intra-ocular portion of the optic nerve – the optic disc – is termed *papillitis,* while involvement of the nerve posterior to the optic disc is termed *retrobulbar neuritis.* In both conditions visual loss may be severe.

In papillitis the optic disc is swollen and has to be distinguished from papilloedema (page 59); after long-standing papillitis the swollen disc becomes atrophic and pale.

In retrobulbar optic neuritis the optic disc may initially appear normal, but pallor caused by optic atrophy invariably follows.

126 Papillitis. The appearance of the optic disc is similar to that found in papilloedema, but visual acuity is severely affected.

Optic atrophy

Optic atrophy may occur secondary to optic neuritis, optic nerve compression or trauma. The optic disc appears pale on fundoscopy and, traditionally, three clinical entities are described.

1. *Primary optic atrophy:* the optic disc is pale and flat with the margin well-defined – indicating that there was no preceding optic disc swelling.

2. *Secondary optic atrophy:* occurs after long-standing optic disc swelling due to papillitis or papilloedema; a pale, swollen optic disc with ill-defined margins results.

3. *Consecutive optic atrophy:* here pallor of the optic disc occurs in association with a primary retinal disorder, e.g. retinitis pigmentosa (page 14).

127 Primary optic atrophy. The optic disc is white and flat and its margin well-defined; the cause is an optic nerve glioma.

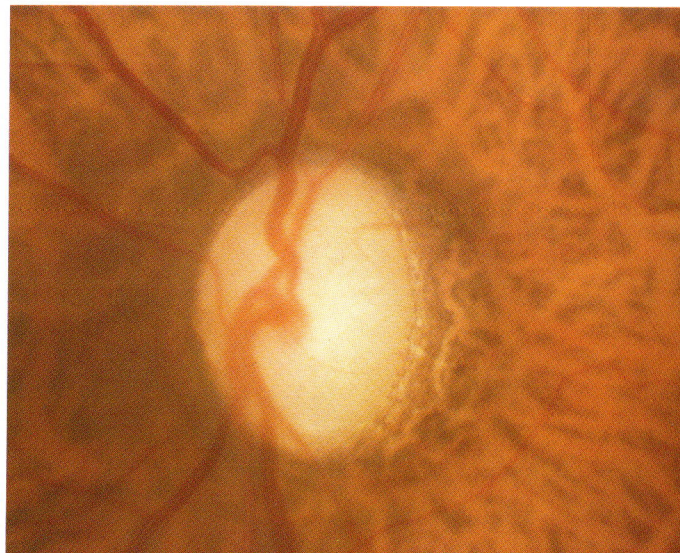

Papilloedema

Papilloedema is a sign of raised intracranial pressure, typically caused by a space-occupying lesion in the posterior cranial fossa. It also presents in association with a number of systemic disorders (hypertension, pulmonary insufficiency, blood dyscrasias) or may be caused by conditions which obstruct the drainage of the central retinal vein (orbital tumours, cavernous sinus thrombosis).

Optic disc swelling is accompanied by loss of retinal vein pulsation and by haemorrhages extending from the optic disc into the adjacent retina. In the early stages vision may be only slightly affected, with some enlargement of the blind spot. However, chronic papilloedema leads to progressive constriction of the peripheral field, loss of vision, and secondary optic atrophy.

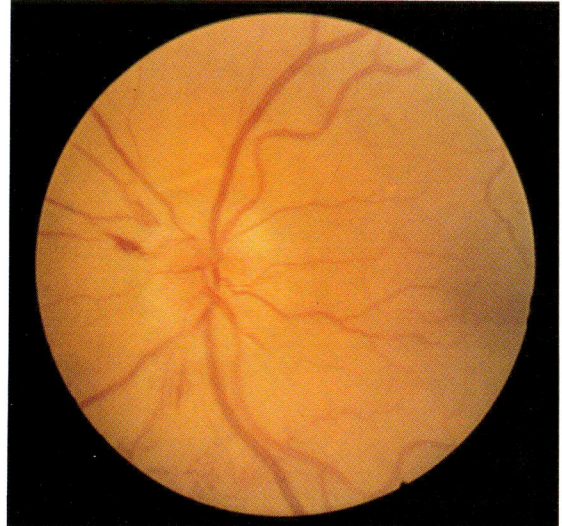

128 Papilloedema of the optic disc. The disc margin and cup are ill-defined due to congestion.

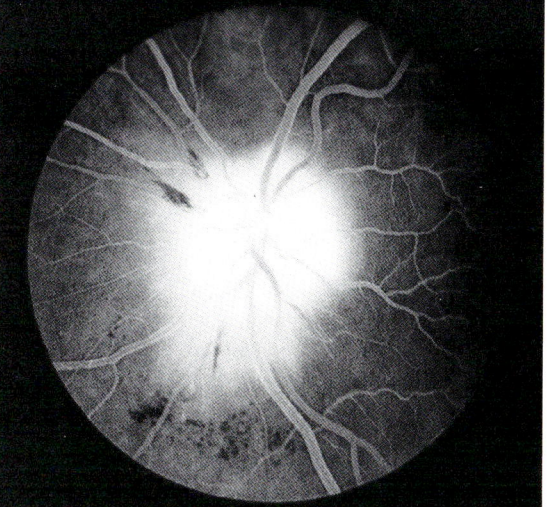

129 Fluorescein angiogram of papilloedema. Profuse leakage of dye from the vessels of the optic disc is a characteristic feature.

PHAKOMATOSES

The term phakomatoses originates from the Greek word 'phakos' meaning 'birth mark' and is used to describe a group of congenital ectodermal dysplasias, typically hamartomas, characterised by abnormalities of the nervous system, skin, eyes and other organs.

Five different syndromes are currently recognised:

Neurofibromatosis (von Recklinghausen's disease)
Tuberous sclerosis (Bourneville's disease)
Cerebelloretinal haemangioblastomatosis (von Hippel-Lindau disease)
Encephalotrigeminal angiomatosis (Sturge-Weber syndrome)
Ataxia telangiectasia (Louis-Bar syndrome).

Neurofibromatosis (von Recklinghausen's disease)

Neurofibromatosis originates as a developmental defect of neurectoderm, probably neural crest, and is transmitted as an autosomal dominant trait.

Pigmented skin lesions ('café-au-lait spots') and multiple neurofibromas occur in association with widespread tumours and other systemic manifestations.

Almost all of the structures of the eye may be affected, either directly or indirectly, often as the result of pressure effects of tumours in other sites. Ocular manifestations of neurofibromatosis include the following:

Orbit: proptosis, which may be the result of erosion of the orbital fissures by meningioma and which may transmit pulsations from the internal carotid artery;
Eyelids: ptosis (plexiform neuroma of the eyelid), 'café-au-lait spots', lagophthalmos (failure of closure) caused by facial nerve damage by acoustic neuroma
Globe: enlargement of the eye (buphthalmos) caused by congenital glaucoma
Cornea: corneal exposure from lagophthalmos (facial nerve damage) and corneal anaesthesia (trigeminal nerve damage) – both caused by acoustic neuroma; thickening of the corneal nerves (visible only by slitlamp biomicroscopy)

Conjunctiva: plexiform neuromas
Iris: neurofibromas
Retina: astrocytomas ('mulberry tumours')
Optic nerve: glioma, meningioma, optic atrophy, papilloedema, optic disc drusen, myelination of the optic disc.

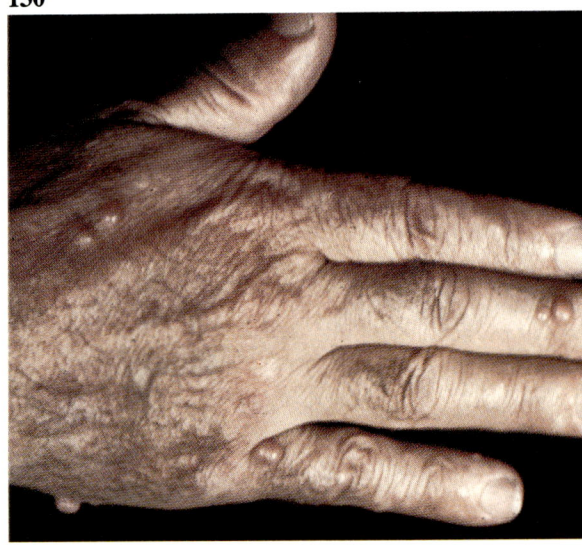

130 Neurofibromatosis of the hand, showing multiple fibromas.

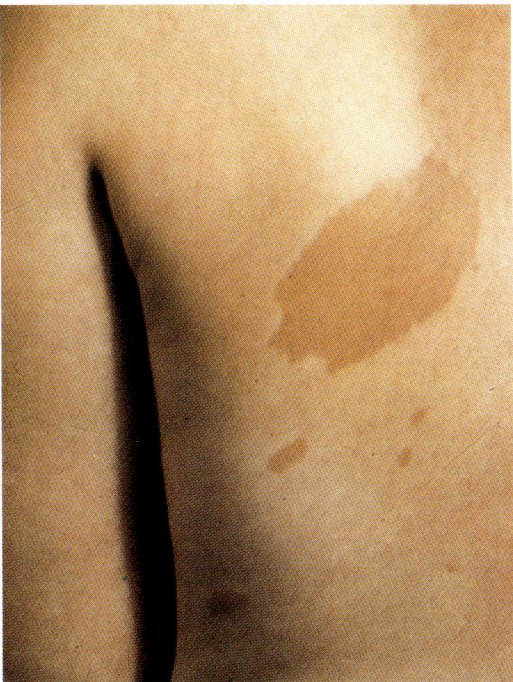

131 'Café-au-lait spots'. Multiple skin lesions should alert to the diagnosis of neurofibromatosis.

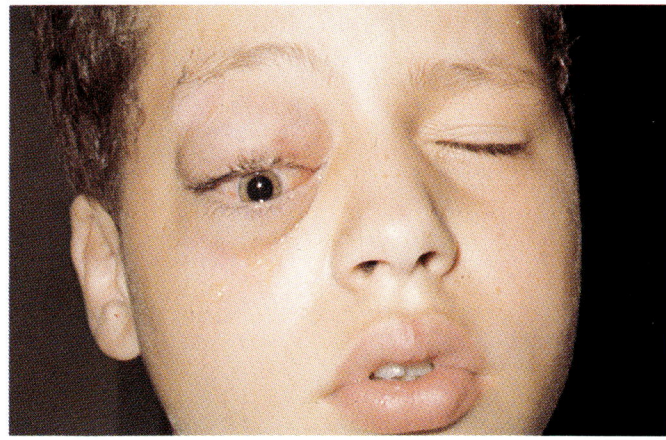

132 Proptosis. The right eye is displaced by a glioma of the optic nerve.

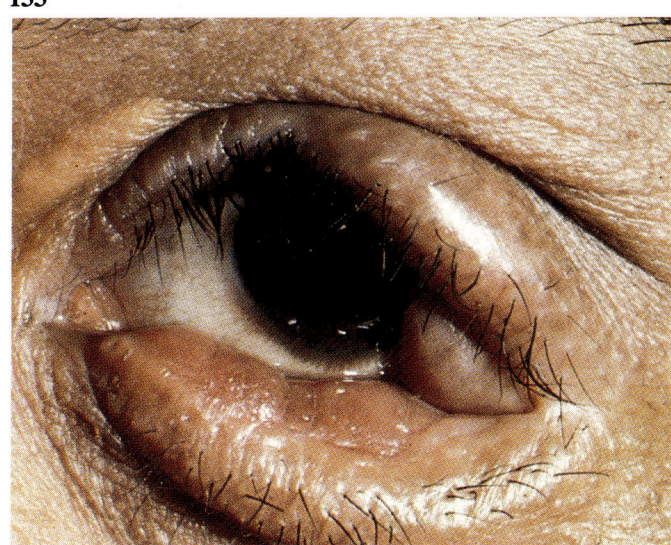

133 Plexiform neuroma deforms the eyelids in neurofibromatosis. (The xanthelasmata are a coincidental finding.)

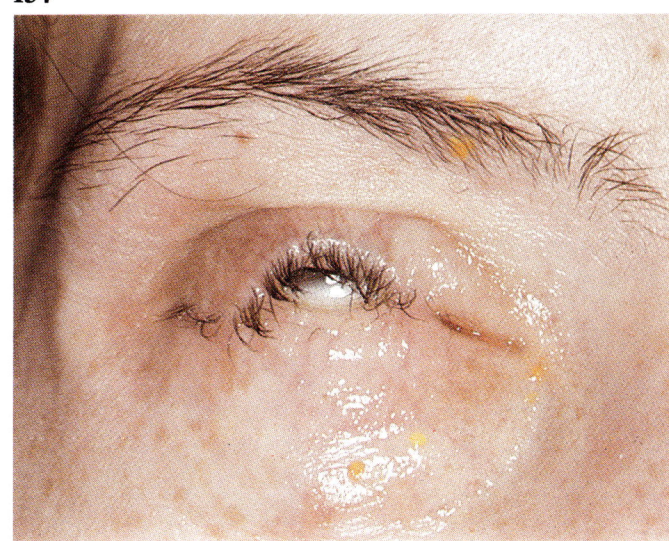

134 Exposure of the cornea caused by lagophthalmos has resulted in corneal scarring. Tarsorrhaphy (suturing of the eyelids) has been performed to aid their closure. (Illustration by courtesy of Mr M J Roper-Hall.)

135 Neurofibromas of the iris. The tumours have formed small brown nodules on the surface of the iris.

136 An astrocytoma of the retina appears as a pale, multi–lobular 'mulberry tumour' in the fundus.

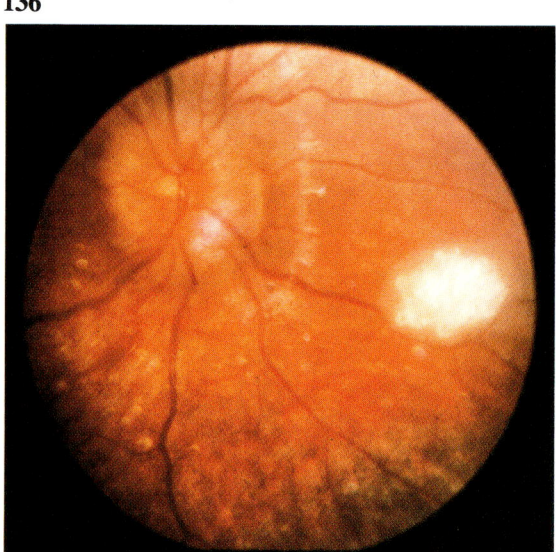

137 Myelination of the optic disc occurs more frequently in cases of neurofibromatosis than in the general population. The affected fibres are shiny white with feathery margins and typically obscure the underlying retinal vessels.

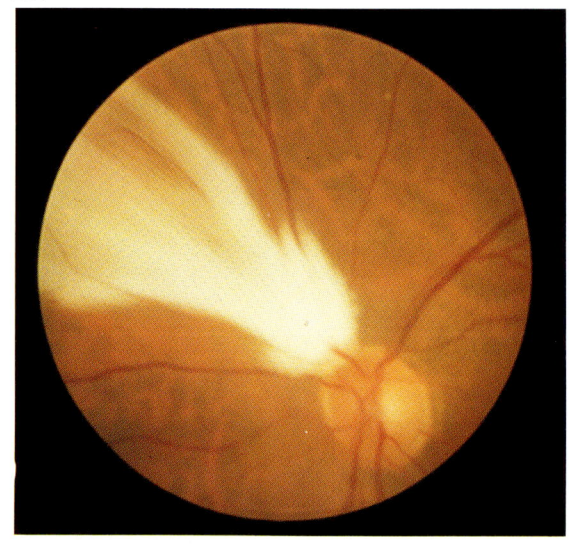

Tuberous sclerosis (Bourneville's disease)

This disorder is characterised by the clinical triad of adenoma sebaceum, mental deficiency and epilepsy; it is inherited as an autosomal dominant trait. Multiple hamartomas occur in the brain, retina and viscera.

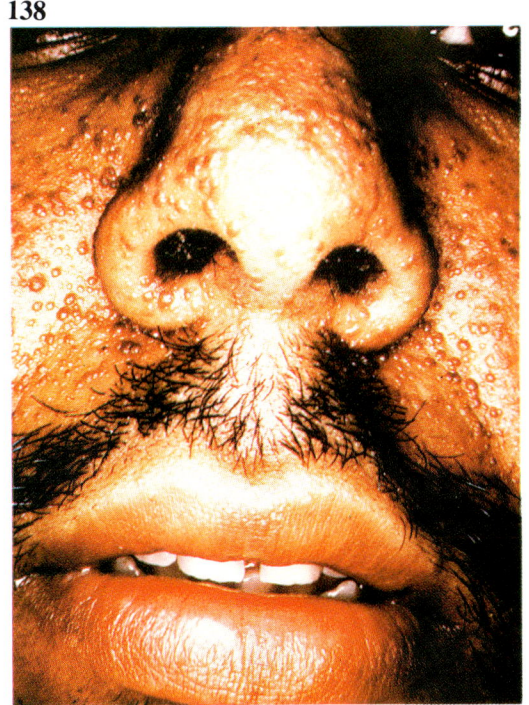

138 Adenoma sebaceum. Small wart-like lesions are scattered in a typical 'butterfly' pattern over the cheeks and nose.

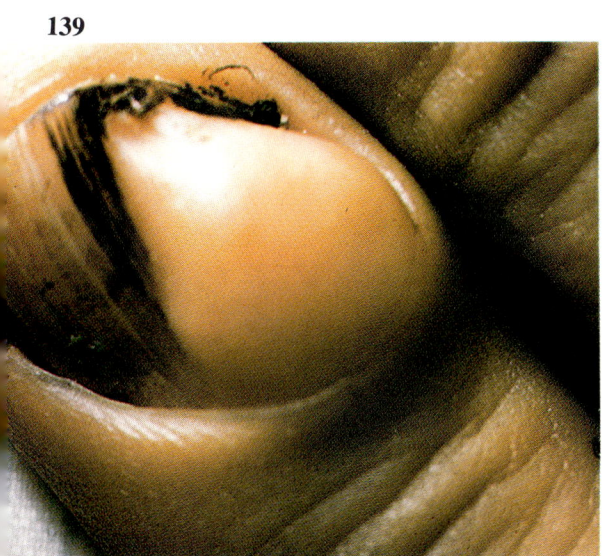

139 Subungual fibroma. This lesion is pathognomic of tuberous sclerosis.

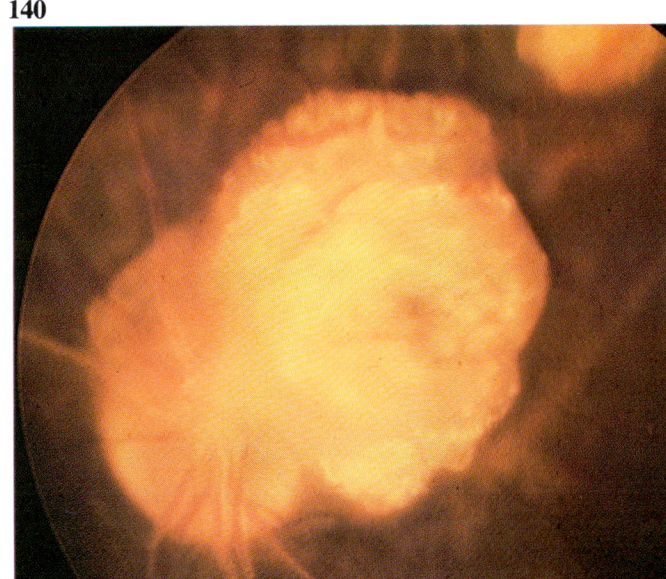

140 Tuberous sclerosis with a glistening multi-lobulated mulberry-like astrocytoma involving the optic disc and adjacent retina.

Cerebelloretinal haemangioblastomatosis (von Hippel-Lindau disease)

In this disorder, angioblastic tumours of the retina are associated with haemangioblastomas of the cerebellum and viscera. Involvement of the kidney may lead to polycythaemia, possibly as the result of increased production of erythropoeitin. The condition may be transmitted as an autosomal dominant character, but most cases arise spontaneously.

A dilated and tortuous feeding artery and draining vein may be the most readily visible sign of a retinal angioma in the peripheral fundus. Increasing size and fluid exudation may lead to the 'exaggerated macular response' or an extensive exudative retinal detachment. Secondary glaucoma with destruction of the eye may follow.

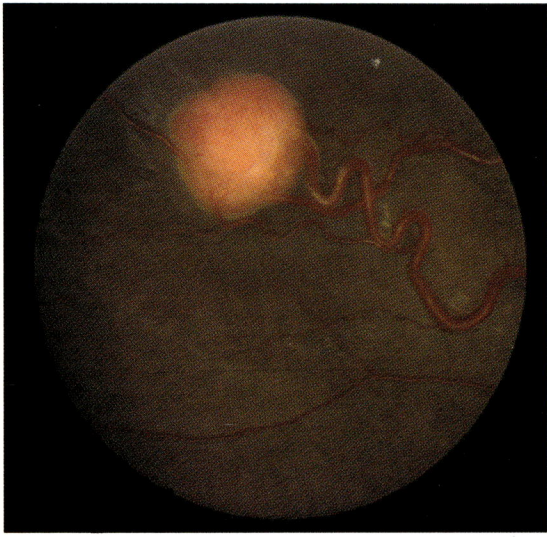

141 Peripheral retinal angioma indicated by the presence of a prominently dilated and tortuous feeding artery and draining vein.

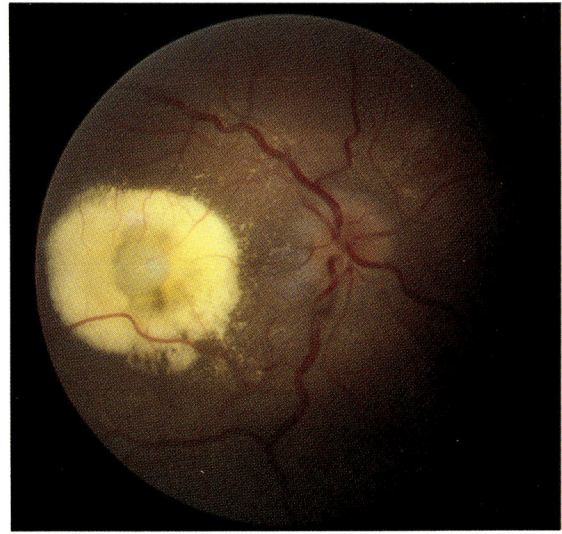

142 Exaggerated macular response. As exudation from the angioma increases, fluid accumulates in the macula.

Encephalotrigeminal angiomatosis (Sturge-Weber syndrome)

In this non-familial disorder, capillary or cavernous haemangiomas occur in the skin of the face in the dermatome supplied by the trigeminal nerve (naevus flammeus). Intracranial haemangiomas in the leptomeninges are associated with 'coral-like' calcification of the underlying cerebral cortex, seizure disorders and mental retardation.

Ocular manifestations include haemangiomas of the eyelids, conjunctiva, episclera, iris and choroid. Involvement of the upper eyelid is commonly associated with tumours of the episclera which cause congenital glaucoma and enlargement of the eye (buphthalmos). Secondary cataract formation and optic atrophy may also occur later.

143 Sturge-Weber syndrome with a typical 'port wine stain' involving the face.

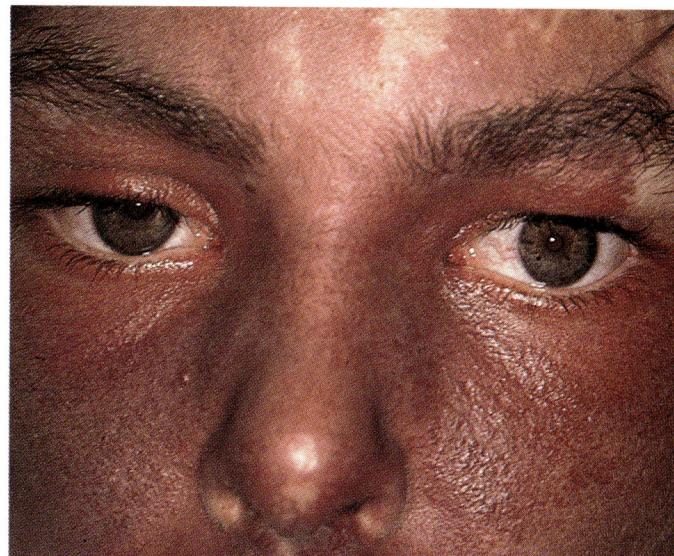

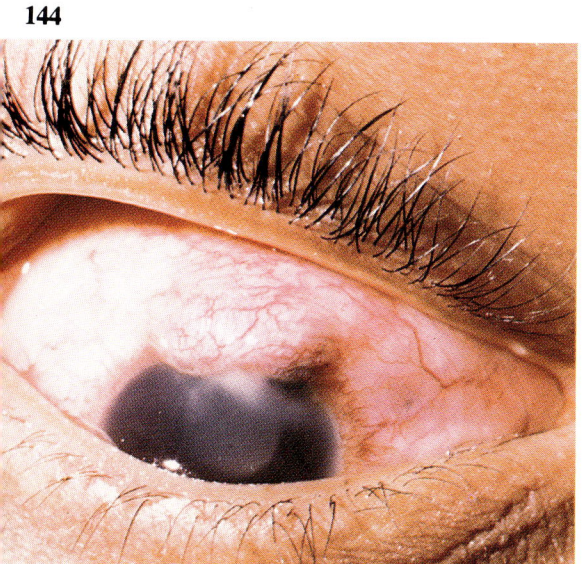

144 Haemangioma of the conjunctiva and underlying episclera.

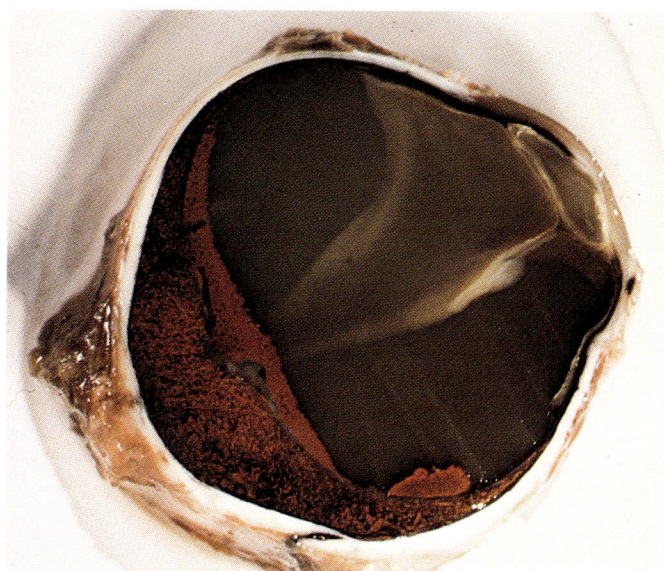

145 Choroidal haemangioma. This postmortem specimen shows a dark red vascular tumour in the posterior pole of the eye; the eye is enlarged (buphthalmos) and the sclera thinned because of congenital glaucoma. A secondary retinal detachment is present.

Ataxia – telangiectasia (Louis-Bar syndrome)

This autosomal recessive disorder may involve the skin, central nervous system, haematopoietic and lymphoreticular systems, and the eye. It is characterised by progressive cerebellar ataxia, telangiectatic lesions of the skin and conjunctiva, and generalised immunological incompetence. Because of the deficiencies in IgA and delayed hypersensitivity, recurrent infections result in early death.

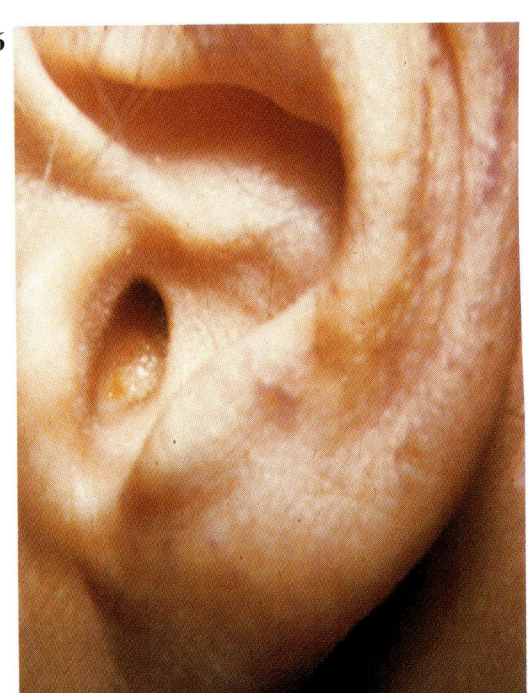

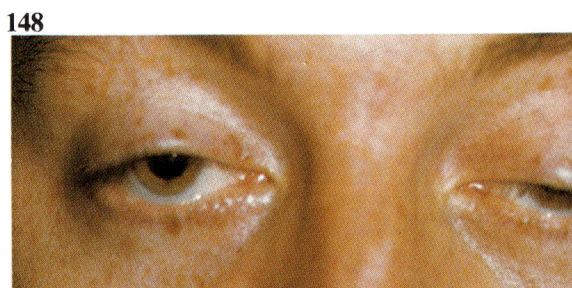

147 Conjunctival telangiectasia typically involves only the globe and not the tarsal conjunctiva.

146 Telangiectases on the ear. They may also occur in the flexor skin areas of the elbows, knees and neck.

MUSCLE DISORDERS
Myasthenia gravis

This chronic disorder of neuromuscular transmission is characterised by progressive muscle weakness and a tendency to tire easily. The ocular, facial, oropharyngeal and respiratory muscles, all of which are controlled by cranial nerves, are especially involved.

The diagnosis is based upon a history of rapid muscle fatigue on repeated exertion and confirmed by the recovery of muscle power following intravenous injection of the cholinergic drug edrophonium.

Ocular manifestations of ptosis and ophthalmoplegia with diplopia may be the presenting features; the ptosis is usually bilateral but asymmetrical.

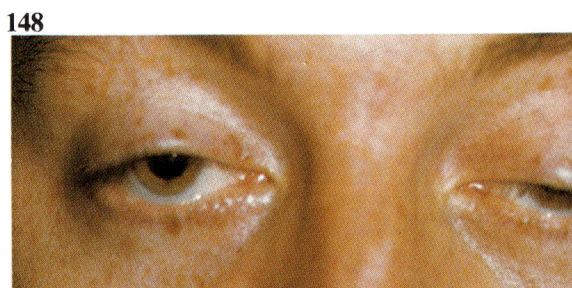

148 Ptosis in myasthenia gravis (before injection of edrophonium).

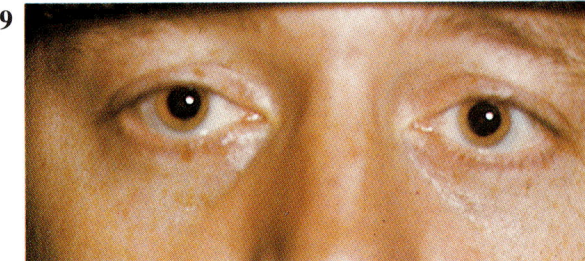

149 Recovery of ptosis after injection of edrophonium.

Myotonic dystrophy

In this rare and complex disorder, muscular dystrophy is progressive and leads to weakness and wasting of the limbs and of the sternomastoid and facial muscles. The myotonia, consisting of delayed muscle relaxation after voluntary contraction, gives rise to a characteristically prolonged grip and handshake. Other features of the disorder include frontal baldness, cardiomyopathy, mental deterioration, late gonadal atrophy and other endocrine abnormalities. When fertile, individuals transmit the disease as a dominant character.

Ocular abnormalities comprise ptosis, pigmentary retinal dystrophy and a star-shaped cataract which is pathognomic.

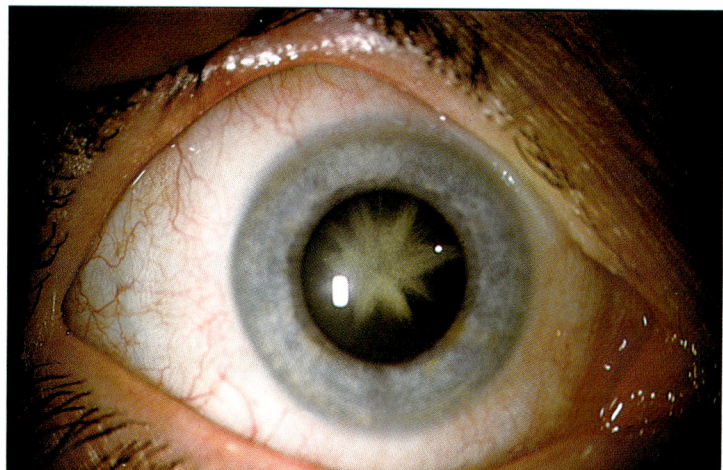

150 Cataract in myotonic dystrophy. The characteristic stellate opacity is situated in the posterior lens capsule.

Index

Figures in light type refer to pages; those in **bold** type refer to illustrations and/or legends.

Abetalipoproteinaemia, 14, 57, **13, 14**
Acne rosacea, 37, 38, **79, 80**
Acromegaly, 41, **85-87**
Addison's disease, 40
Adenoma sebaceum, 63, **138**
Albinism, 9, 10, **4, 5**
Amaurosis fugax, 25, 54, **105**
Anaemia, 53, 57, **116**
Angioid streaks, 16, **18**
Angioma, 64, **141**
Ankylosing spondylitis, 19
Arachnodactyli, **15**
Arcus senilis, *see Corneal arcus*
Astrocytoma, 60, **136, 140**
Ataxia telangiectasia, 60, 66, **146, 147**
Atopic eczema, 37, **76-78**

Bacterial infections, 27-8, **49-52**
Bacterial septicaemia, 27, **49, 50**
Bassen-Kornzweig syndrome, 14, **13, 14**
Behçet's syndrome, 19, 26, **46-48**
Bengal rose dye test, **28**
Bitot spots, 57, **124**
Blepharitis, **80**
Blood (hyperviscosity) 54, **117**
Bourneville's disease, 60, 63, **138-140**
Buphthalmos, 64, **145**

'Café-au-lait spots', 60, **131**
Candida albicans, **64, 65**
Carcinoma (bronchial), 51, **111-113**

Cataract
– in congenital rubella, 30, **57**
– in diabetes mellitus, 44, **95**
– in galactosaemia ('oil drop'), 11, **6**
– in herpes zoster ophthalmicus, 31, **62**
– iatrogenic, **32**
– in myotonic dystrophy ('star-shaped'), 67, **150**
– in Wilson's disease ('sunflower'), 9, **2**
Cerebelloretinal haemangioblastomatosis, 60, 64, **141, 142**
'Cherry-red spot', **104**
Chloroquine retinopathy, **42**
Chorioretinitis (in syphilis), 29, **54**
Choroid (haemangioma), 64, **145**
Choroidal circulation (fovea), **104**
Choroidal metastasis, 51, **112**
Coats' disease, 12, **13**
Conjunctiva
– Bitot spot, 57, **124**
– fibrosis (cicatricial), **82**
– haemangioma, 64, **144**
– infiltration (Hodgkin's disease), 56, **122**
– jaundice, **125**
– oedema, 42, **90, 91**
– telangiectasia, 18, **23**
– vascular dilatation, 42, **77, 89**
Conjunctivitis
– in measles, 30, **56**
– in Reiter's syndrome, **36**
– in Stevens-Johnson syndrome, 39, **82**
Cornea
– calcification, 52, **114**
– exposure and scarring, 31, 39, **26, 53, 61, 83, 134**
– infiltration (acne rosacea), **80**
– keratic precipitates ('mutton fat'), **72, 73**
– necrosis, **49**
– ulcer, **77**
– – dendritic, **115**
Corneal arcus, 12, **8**
'Cotton wool spots', 48, **40, 99, 103, 116**
Cranial nerves
– fifth (trigeminal)
– – in encephalotrigeminal angiomatosis, 64, **143**
– – in herpes zoster ophthalmicus, 31, **59**
– fourth (trochlear), 41, 58
– sixth (abducens)
– – palsy, 41, **87**

– third (oculomotor)
– – palsy, 31, 41, 44, **60, 93**
Crohn's disease, 57
Cushing's disease, 40
Cyanotic congenital heart disease, 50, **107-109**
Cysticercosis, 34, **69**

Dermatomyositis, 19
Diabetes mellitus, 44, **93-102**
Diabetic retinopathy, 44
– advanced, **101**
– background, **96**
– maculopathy, **98**
– pre-proliferative, **99**
– proliferative, **97, 100, 102**

Ectopia lentis
– in homocystinuria, 10, **3**
– in Marfan's syndrome, 15, **16**
Ehlers-Danlos syndrome, 15, 17, **19-21**
Encephalotrigeminal angiomatosis, 60, 64, **143-145**
Endophthalmitis
– fungal, 33, **64**
– septic, 27, **49**
Enophthalmia, **111**
Episclera (haemangioma), 64, **144**
Episcleritis, 19, **29**
Erythema
– in acne rosacea, 38, **79**
– in atopic eczema, 76, **77**
– in systemic lupus erythematosus, **39**
Erythema multiforme, *see Stevens-Johnson syndrome*
Exophthalmos, *see Proptosis*
Extra-ocular muscles
– lateral rectus, **87, 89,** *see also Cranial nerves, Proptosis*
Exudates (retinal)
– hard, **96, 98, 103**
– soft, *see 'Cotton wool spots'*

Fibroma, **130**
– subungal, **139**
Fluorescein angiography, **97, 120, 129**
Fluorescein stain (corneal ulcer), **77, 115**
Fovea ('cherry-red spot'), **104**
Friedrickson (classification, hyperlipidaemia). 12
Fungal infections, 33, **64-67**

Galactosaemia, 9, 11, 52, **6**
Giant cell arteritis, 19, 25, **43, 44**
Glaucoma
– congenital (buphthalmos), 64, **145**
– neovascular, 44, **94**
– secondary, **72**
Gout, 19, 23, **37, 38**
Granulomas, *see Sarcoidosis*
Grave's disease, 42, **88-92**
Grönblad-Strandberg syndrome, 15, 16, **17, 18**

Haemangioma
– of choroid, **145**
– of conjunctiva and episclera, **144**
Haemorrhage (systemic), 18, 57, *see also Retinal vascular abnormalities*
Hamartomas, *see Phakomatoses*
Hepatolenticular degeneration, 9, **1, 2**
Herpes simplex (dendritic ulcer), 52, **115**
Herpes zoster ophthalmicus, 31, 37, **59-63**
'Histo spots', 33, **67**
Histoplasmosis (Histoplasmosis capsulatum), 33, **66, 67**
Hodgkin's disease, 56, **122**
Homocystinuria, 9, 10, 52, **3**
Horner's syndrome, **111**
Hutchinson's sign, **59**
Hutchinson's triad, **53**
Hyperlipidaemia, 9, 12, 57, **7-12**
Hyperparathyroidism, 40
Hyperphosphataemia, 52, **114**
Hypertension (systemic), 48, 52, **103**
Hypocalcaemia, 52

Hypoparathyroidism, 40
Hypopyon, **47**
Hypothalamus (suprasellar tumours), 40

Iatrogenic complications,
– chloroquine, **42**
– systemic steroids, 52, **32, 115**
Iridocyclitis, 19, 22, **34, 35**
Iris
– atrophy, 31, **62**
– iridodinesis, **16**
– metastasis, 51, **113**
– neurofibromas, 60, **135**
see also Rubeosis iridis
Iritis
– ciliary injection, **38, 72**
– in gout, 23, 52, **38**
– severe recurring, **47**

Jaundice, **125**

Kayser-Fleischer ring, 9, **1**
Keratitis (interstitial), **53**
Keratoconjunctivitis, **80**
Keratoconjunctivitis sicca, 19, 20, **26-28**
Keratoconus, **78**
Keratopathy
– calcific band, 19, 22, **35**
– lipid, 12, **9**

Lacrimal gland infiltration, 35, **71**
Laser, *see Photocoagulation*
Laurence-Moon-Biedl syndrome, 14, **13, 14**
Lens (dislocation), 10, 15, **3, 16,** *see also* Cataract

Leukaemia, 56, **121, 123**
Lipaemia retinalis, 12, **10**
Louis-Bar syndrome, 60, 66, **146, 147**

Macula ('bull's-eye'), **42**
Macular
– haemorrhage, **66**
– response ('exaggerated'), 64, **142**
– scar, 16, **18**
– 'star', **103**
Maculopathy (diabetic), **98**
Malabsorption syndrome, 57
Marfan's syndrome, 15, **15, 16**
Metastases (bronchial carcinoma), 51, **112, 113**
Microphthalmos (congenital rubella), 30, **57**
Miosis (Horner's syndrome), **111**
Multiple hereditary haemorrhagic
  telangiectasia, 18, **22-24**
Myasthenia gravis, 58, 66, **148, 149**
Myotonic dystrophy, 58, 67, **150**
Myxoedema, 40

Naevus flammeus, 64, **143**
Neurofibroma, 60, **135**
Neurofibromatosis, 60, **130-137**
Neuroma, 60, **133**

Oedema
– periorbital and facial, 34, **70**
– retinal, **104**
Optic atrophy, 41, 58, 59, **55, 86, 127**
Optic chiasma (compression), 41
Optic disc
– astrocytoma, **140**
– in ischaemic optic neuropathy, **44**
– myelination, 60, **137**
– neovascularisation, **75, 97, 100**
see also Optic atrophy, Papillitis, Papilloedema
Optic neuritis, 58

Papillitis, 58, **126**
Papilloedema, 58, 59, **128, 129**
– in respiratory insufficiency, 50, **110**
– in systemic hypertension, 48, **103**
Parasitic infections, 34, **68-70**
Phakomatoses, 58, 60, **130-147**
Pheochromocytoma, 40
Photocoagulation (diabetic retinopathy), **102**
Phytanic acid storage disease, 14, **13, 14**
Pituitary (anterior lobe) tumours, 41, **85-87**
Polycythaemia, 54, **109, 117**
Polymyositis, 19
Progressive systemic sclerosis, 19
Proptosis
– in Grave's disease, 42, **90, 91**
– in leukaemia, 56, **121**
– in neurofibromatosis, 60, **132**
– in posterior scleritis, **31**
Pseudoxanthoma elasticum, 16, **17**
Psoriatic arthropathy, 19
Ptosis
– in Horner's syndrome, **111**
– in myasthenia gravis, 66, **148, 149**
– third nerve palsy, 31, 44, **60, 93**
Pupil
– miosis, **111**
– posterior synechiae, **34, 38**

Refsum's disease, 14, **13, 14**
Reiter's syndrome, 19, 23, **36**
Renal
– failure, 52, **114**
– transplant (complications), 52, **115**
Rendu-Osler-Weber syndrome, 15, 18, 57, **22-24**
Respiratory insufficiency, 50, **110**
Retina
– angioid streaks, 16, **18**
– angioma, 64, **141**
– astrocytoma, 60, **136, 140**
– cyanosis, 50, **109**
– detachment, **52, 101, 145**
– leukaemic infiltration, 56, **123**
– scarring
– – panphotocoagulation, **102**
– – retinochoroiditis, **68**

Retinal vascular abnormalities
– haemorrhage
– – in blood dyscrasias, 53-54, **116, 118**
– – in diabetic retinopathy, **96, 97**
– – macular, **66**
– inflammation (posterior ciliary arteries), **44**
– ischaemia, 48, **40, 97, 103**
– microaneurysms, **96, 97**
– morphological changes, 48, **99, 103, 104, 110, 117, 118, 141,** see also Lipaemia retinalis
– neovascularisation, **75, 97, 100, 119, 120**
– occlusion
– – arterial, 48, **11, 45, 104, 105**
– – venous, 48, 49, **48, 75, 106**
– – and necrosis, **63**
– periphlebitis, **48, 74, 75**
– telangiectasia, 18, **12, 24**
– vasculitis (obliterative), **41**
Retinitis
– candida albicans, **64, 65**
– necrotising, 34, **68**
– pigmentosa, 9, 14, **13, 14**
– in rubella, 30, **58**
Retinochoroiditis (Toxoplasmosis), 34, **68**
Retinopathy
– chloroquine, **42**
– in sickle cell disease, 54, **118-120**
see also Diabetic retinopathy
Retrobulbar neuritis, 58
Rheumatic fever, 19
Rheumatoid arthritis, 19, 20, **25-32,** see also Still's disease
Rhinophyma, 38, **79**
Roth spots, **50, 116**
Rubella, 30, **57, 58**
Rubeola, 30, **56**
Rubeosis iridis, 44, **94**

'Salmon patch' (sickle cell disease), 54, **118**
Sarcoidosis, 35, **71-75**
Schirmer's test, **27**
Sclera
– blueing, 17, **21**
– jaundice, **125**
Scleritis, 19, **30**
Scleroderma, 19

Scleromalacia perforans, **30**
'Sea fan' (sickle cell disease), 54, **119, 120**
Sickle cell disease, 54, **118-120**
Sjögren's syndrome, 20, **26-28, 71**
Spirochaetal infection, *see Syphilis*
Squint (congenital rubella), **57**
Stevens-Johnson syndrome, 38-39, **81-84**
Still's disease, 19, 22, **33-35**
Sturge-Weber syndrome, 60, 64, **143-145**
Subungual fibroma, **139**
Symblepharon, 39, **84**
Synechiae (posterior), **34, 38**
Syphilis, 29, **53-55**
Systemic lupus erythematosus, 19, 24, **39-42**

Taenia solium, *see Cysticercosis*
Takayasu's disease, 19, 25, **45**
Tarsorrhaphy, **61, 92, 134**
Telangiectasia, 18
– conjunctival **23, 147**
– – and corneal, **80**
– facial, 38, **22, 79, 146**
– retinal, **12, 24**
Toxoplasmosis (Toxoplasmosis gondii), 34, **68**
Trichinosis (Trichinella spiralis), 34, **70**
Tuberculosis, 28, **51, 52**
Tuberous sclerosis, 60, 63, **138-140**
Tumours
– pituitary (anterior lobe), 41, **85-87**
– suprasellar, 40
see also Phakomatoses

Ulcerative colitis, 57
Usher's syndrome, 14, **13, 14**
Uveitis
– anterior, *see Iritis*
– posterior, *see Chorioretinitis*

Varicella, 31
Vasculitis, 19
– obliterative, **41**
Viral infections, 30-31, **56-63**
Vitamin deficiencies, 9, 57, **124**
von Hippel-Lindau disease, 52, 60, 64, **141, 142**
von Recklinghausen's disease, 60, **130-137**

Wegener's granulomatosis, 19
Wilson's disease, 9, 52, 57, **1, 2**

Xanthelasmata, 12, **7, 133**

Zoster, *see Herpes zoster ophthalmicus*

RC
73
.5
K73
1984
c.2
OPTO